My Brain Implant for Bionic Vision

This Page Intentionally Left Blank

My Brain Implant for Bionic Vision

The First Trial of Artificial Sight for the Blind

Richard B. McDonald
www.richardbmcdonald.com

Dedication

To my beautiful and amazing wife Charina
without whose love and support
I would not have had the courage to volunteer
into this first-ever clinical trial of a
brain implant for bionic vision.
"The Wonder of You" - A song by Elvis Presley

This Page Intentionally Left Blank

Table of Contents

Chapter 1 - Before the Brain Implant for Bionic Vision

Among the most scary and depressing days in my life was when my eye doctor told me that, "Your eye is not salvageable." That was about 13 years ago when I was 40. The doctor was talking about my left eye. He said this after a couple of years of trying everything known to mankind at that time to save my eyesight: valve implants into the eye, corneal transplants, laser treatments and on and on and on. I had already gone blind in my right eye a decade earlier. So, this meant that I was Now totally and permanently blind. The doctor was not being unkind or insensitive. Instead, he was just being matter-of-fact. I can only imagine how difficult it must be for a doctor to say such a thing to another human being.

This all happened to me at the Jules Stein Eye Institute at the University of California at Los Angeles (UCLA). My response to this doctor 13 years ago was, "Well, you guys had better get busy down in the lab and figure something out." And then, among the most happy and hopeful days in my life was when in mid-2018 I got a phone call from UCLA saying that I had been accepted into the first-ever clinical trial for a brain implant for bionic vision. Lo and behold - the good doctors at UCLA had indeed figured something out! This book carries the most amazing story of this happy and hopeful happening.

The greatest news is that this happening is not just for me but, rather, maybe for you too, maybe for one of your friends or maybe for one of your family members. And, maybe none of those people have eye trouble presently, but they might one day in the future. Maybe they are not even born yet? It does not even matter why they lost their eyesight because this bionic vision completely bypasses all of the mechanisms of the eye and goes straight to the brain. One thing is for sure, there is now hope for millions and millions of people around the world who are or who may become blind.

In this chapter, I want to tell you why I volunteered for this. At the end of this chapter, I will give some background on how I lost my eyesight. In the next and subsequent chapters, I will talk about the clinical trial for a brain implant for bionic vision and the bionic laboratory. The remainder of this book relays the story of coming home with bionic vision, societal considerations connected with bionics and concludes with what the future may hold for bionic vision. In that final chapter, some of the early work on bionic vision will be discussed. Naturally, as far-out as the Orion is, like all technological advancements it has built on decades and decades of earlier work.

I should also say here that I am on a life-long journey. The clinical trial of the Orion brain implant for bionic vision in which I am participating is a five-year study. At the time of this book's publication (2019), I am only about a year into it. You can visit my website at richardbmcdonald.com where I will blog about the evolution of the Orion and my own process of learning to see again. The technologies involved here, as well as my own process of learning to see again, are continuously evolving. Nobody knows how far this will go.

Very clearly I say that everything in this book are my own, personal experiences, thoughts and opinions. No person, corporation or institution ever made any predictions, suggestions or promises about what may or may not result from going through with this. To the contrary, every person, corporation and institution cautioned me rigorously about all the risks and no-expectations nature involved here. This caveat extends to every person, corporation like Second Sight and institution like UCLA mentioned in this book. With that, now let me tell you why I did it.

Why I Did It

When I lost my eyesight 13 years ago all my friends and family said, "Well, Richie, maybe someday they will develop a bionic eye." At the beginning of 2018 I lay in bed pondering how I could possibly, logistically or financially, travel the world to discover what might be out there for me. This seemed to be an impossible thing to do since I am not wealthy. And, being blind, it is not possible simply to head-out globe trekking by myself. Like every disabled person, I forever dream of one day, somehow, regaining my lost ability. For me, it is eyesight. For others, it is walking, hearing or whatever.

I had heard wisps in the wind of stem cells, drugs and even faith-healers. Perhaps there was something in China or Europe or even a guru atop a mountain in India. Maybe there was a faith healer in Brazil? I had even heard of bionic vision work being done in Australia. Maybe there was *something* for me, I thought. After all, 13 years had passed since I went blind. Indeed, the iPhone had not even been introduced then!

So, one reason I volunteered into this clinical trial is that *it came to me*. That is, I did not have to go on a global quest searching for eyesight. This trial of a brain implant for bionic vision (called the Orion) would be conducted at UCLA. I live 15 minutes away from UCLA! So, I did not need to go anywhere! As you will read in the next chapter, the Orion is the most advanced, far-out scientific and medical technology on the planet. It holds the best, most perfect chance for me to regain eyesight. I would receive the very best care and attention imaginable.

Not to be overlooked, this would all come to me for free! Even if the Orion were presently commercially available, for what I would receive in the trial, it would cost millions of dollars. None of this would be covered by medical insurance. It is, at this point, experimental. Can anyone imagine any greater gift? Of course, by the time the Orion becomes commercially available, it will not cost millions of dollars, but it will not be cheap either. However, by then medical insurance is likely to cover it.

Another reason to do it was that I thought "If not me, then who?" That is, humankind could benefit beyond comprehension from something like a cure for blindness. I really had a chance to do something fantastic for us all, both presently and for us all in the future. How many among us get such a glorious opportunity in life? Well, somebody has to go first, right? I will do it. And, you can all count on me to do my level-best.

I also thought I had the "right stuff." I have always wanted to be an explorer way out on the frontier. There is a movie called <u>The Right Stuff</u> (1987) about the first astronauts. It's about them having what it would take to go where no one had gone before - space. It's about being on the very cutting edge of the world's technology. It's about exploring the unknown. And finally, it is about doing something for the benefit of humanity. To me, this whole Orion thing sounded pretty exciting, cool and maybe even fun.

Not a trivial consideration of whether to do it was the hope for regaining some sort of eyesight. Now, not to get too carried away here, I was not under any delusions about the level or kind of vision I might get. I fully understood the rudimentary, synthetic nature of it. Indeed, I was aware that the Orion might not even work at all. In fact, I thought long and hard about the chance that this whole thing could turn me into a vegetable, I could die on the operating table, I could get a brain infection or any other number of serious and dangerous complications. If nothing else, implant brain surgery sort of sounded like it might hurt a little!

I also had to consider my age (52) and the state of my health versus what technological or medical opportunities might be in the future for potentially regaining some eyesight. On the one hand, presently my health is good. But what might happen to me in 10 or 15 years? If I waited, would I be in good enough health if and when something else became available? I figured I could, at most, look-out about 15 years into my late 60s and expect decent health. On the other hand, would the technology or medical capabilities improve in any significant way within this 15-year horizon as compared to what I had here and now with the Orion? After all, as explained in the final chapter of this book about the future of bionic vision, with the Orion I would in fact be able to take advantage of technological advancements for many years to come. This is because it has some built-in future compatibility. So, at the end of this difficult consideration, I concluded that no time would be better than the present.

Lastly, as a kid growing-up in the 1970s, there was a common thing we would say: "Go for it!" Today, we say "Just do it!" Ultimately I thought to myself, "Well I've had a good ride so far, so if it all ended today I'd be more than OK with it all." With that, I concluded "Let's go for it!"

Allow me to say a word here about the concept of courage. People often say to me regarding volunteering into this experimental clinical trial, "Oh, Richie, you are so brave." No, I am not. For example, I cried like a baby as they wheeled me into the operating room. I did not dive right into this. I pondered it thoroughly. I at many times in this voyage been very scared, am today, and will be in the future. Courage is not an absence of fear. It is the resolve to step forward in the face of it.

Background on How I Became Blind

Without going into the details, I was born with glaucoma in both eyes. Glaucoma causes a withering of vision by cutting the connection between the eye and the brain. That is, glaucoma results in a progressive deterioration of the optic nerve. In my right eye, I could only count fingers up until the age of about 15. After that age, in my right eye I was blind. In my left eye, I had some modest vision before it was lost at the age of 40. Basically, for all of my life the best vision I ever had was what is called "legally blind."

In spite of my poor vision, as an adolescent I played Little League baseball, could read newspaper print up until I was about 25 and even drove a car for a few years in my 30s. All these things I did poorly because of my eyesight. I did graduate from college (*cum laude*), and had a career in accounting. For me, I was not blind from birth, nor was the loss of my eyesight a sudden "lights out" thing. Rather, it was a slow, progressive winding down.

I must say here that I am eternally grateful for having what eyesight I did have. For one thing, to me having perfect eyesight and then suddenly totally losing it (like from an accident or an injury) would be very hard to handle. I had time to adjust. The understanding that someday I might lose my eyesight was ever-present. Another thing is that I feel fortunate to have seen many things: spectacular sunsets, the movie <u>Star Wars</u>, a bird in flight and pretty girls to name just a few. Most of all, shortly before I became totally blind I had a couple of years with my wife, Charina. In my mind, she will forever look 25.

I should mention here that most people with my eye condition are blind by early adolescence. Credit for sustaining what vision I had for as long as it lasted goes to my parents. They moved to Los Angeles when I was about 2 years old specifically for the reason that there they thought I could get the very best medical attention. My parents had lived all over the world before I was born. Living in Los Angeles was not in their plans.

Indeed I did get the best medical attention possible. At birth, the doctors could tell that there was something wrong with my eyes just by looking at them. My first eye surgery was at two months old. Between the ages of 2 and 40 years old I had more than 50 different surgeries on my eyes, took a myriad of eye medications and was under the care of the finest eye doctors - all with the goal of sustaining my eyesight. For decades, I would go to eye checkups where doctors would marvel aloud that I could still see anything at all.

It is certain that only because I was living in Los Angeles in 2018 that I had the opportunity to get bionic vision. Were I not living here, I would not have learned about this. I would not be so close to UCLA to make it even logistically possible to participate in the Orion clinical trial. Both of my parents are long dead now. As usual, my parents were right all along. Thanks mom and dad!

This Page Intentionally Left Blank

Chapter 2 - The First Trial of a Brain Implant for Bionic Vision

One night in late February 2018, I lay awake listening to <u>Coast to Coast AM Radio</u>. More correctly, it was very early in the morning, like 3:00 AM. Being blind for the past 12 years, terrible nighttime insomnia had become a regular thing for me. This is a medical condition that the blind often suffer called "Non-24-hour Sleep-wake Disorder." I was at this time 52 years old.

Suddenly, during a commercial break while listening to <u>Coast to Coast</u>, an advertisement came over the radio seeking volunteers (called "participants") for an experimental clinical trial for the first-ever brain implant for bionic vision. The ad said that the clinical trial would be conducted at the University of California at Los Angeles, (UCLA). It also said that there would only be a total of five participants accepted. A few additional qualifications were listed, which I will get into later in this chapter. But, the main thing was that the participant must have previously had vision and that they are currently blind.

"My God," I thought! "Could this be the impossible dream for which I have prayed?" Of course, any hope for sleep that night was now gone. As a matter of fact, if you know anything about <u>Coast to Coast</u>, I was a little unsure if the ad was for real or part of the <u>Coast to Coast</u> radio program itself. The ad sounded so far-out. A brain implant for bionic vision? Seriously? "Isn't that the sort of thing seen only in the movies," I wondered?

Since I did not catch the phone number the ad stated to call regarding the trial, that morning I began frantically Googling for it. Intuitively, I knew that there must be countless blind people trying to get into the trial. Indeed, later I learned that in fact hundreds of blind people wanted in. My odds of getting in were very slim. Just to have a chance to get in, I must move like lightning, I thought! The idea that I might miss this once-in-a-lifetime chance to regain some eyesight terrified me.

Eventually, that morning I reached a generic voicemail box for Sara Rodriguez. Sara was the coordinator at UCLA for the clinical trial. I left a message for her explaining that I think I might qualify. For the next day or so, I kept my phone in my hands desperately hoping that she would call me. When she did return my call a few days later, I was thrilled to get an appointment at UCLA for an initial consultation. That initial consultation happened in early March 2018. It would start my long, strange trip to bionic vision. But, before I go further about qualifying for the clinical trial, first let me explain a bit about just what this bionic vision is all about.

The Clinical Trial

The clinical trial came about under what is known as the "Breakthrough Device Program." Essentially, under this program, the

Food and Drug Administration (FDA) would cut the red tape to bring forward cutting-edge medical technologies that had a reasonable chance of working, but which would otherwise not be available for decades were they to progress through the FDA's normal procedures. We have all heard of the many, many years it takes for medical treatments such as drugs to come to market because of the very long FDA processes. The Breakthrough Device Program is intent on shortening that process.[1]

In late 2017, the FDA granted Second Sight Medical Products, Inc., full approval to proceed with the first-ever human clinical trial of its "Orion" brain implant for bionic vision. It would be a five-year trial. The trial would be conducted at two sites, Baylor College of Medicine and UCLA. Initially, only five participants would be admitted. This was later expanded to six participants. There are four participants at UCLA (of which I am one) and two at Baylor.

Another aspect of the Orion clinical trial is that it would require a great amount of time and effort on the part of the participant. For one thing, it would last five years. For the first couple of years, approximately weekly visits to "the bionic laboratory" would be required. I will talk about the bionic lab in a later chapter. After

---

[1] For an excellent discussion of the FDA's Breakthrough Device Program, see this link:
https://www.medicaldesignandoutsourcing.com/brain-implant-for-some-blind-people-shows-benefits-of-fdas-breakthrough-device-program/

that, periodic, but less frequent, visits to the bionic lab would be required. No participant would be paid anything at all for being in the trial. So, a major commitment on the part of anyone accepted into the trial was necessary.

The clinical trial would test for the safety and effectiveness of the brain implant and its external hardware on humans. Together, the implant and its external hardware are called the "Orion." Next, this stunning technology will be described.

The Orion

Basically, the Orion consists of two main components: a brain implant and the "device." The device has three basic parts: a pair of glasses that has a camera in it, a video processing unit (VPU) and a cable connected to the VPU with an antenna at the other end. The participant wears the glasses. The camera is a lot like the camera in a smart phone. It is mounted in the bridge of the glasses. This camera streams video to the VPU. Really, the magic happens in this VPU. It has all the software (you could call it an app) for converting the video stream from the camera into electrical impulses. The VPU wirelessly transmits those electrical impulses to the brain implant through the antenna at the end of the cable connected to it. That antenna attaches to a head strap worn by the user. The VPU is about the size of three iPhones stacked one atop the others.[2]

The brain implant itself deserves a bit more description. It is a stunning piece of technology. Mostly, it is made of gold, platinum and other precious metals and exotic materials. Pictured below is a rendering of the implant illustrating its placement inside the skull

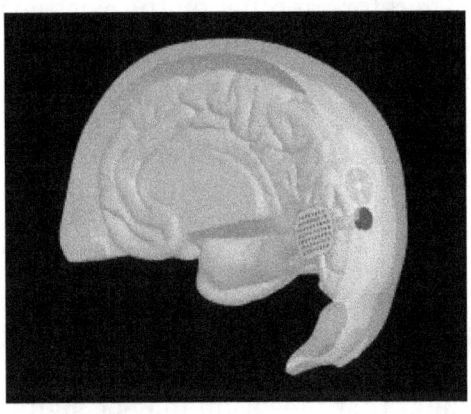

(*source*: MIT Technology Review). The implant has three basic parts: a gold-colored foil about the size of your palm, a very thin cable about three inches long and a microchip about the size of three dimes stacked one atop the others. The gold-colored foil is placed onto the brain's visual cortex. It has 60 electrodes. It is connected to the microchip by the cable. That microchip both receives information from the VPU and sends

---

[2] The MIT Technology Review has an excellent article "Blind Patients to Test Bionic Eye Brain Implants" that gives a more technical explanation of the Orion: https://www.technologyreview.com/s/608844/blind-patients-to-test-bionic-eye-brain-implants/

information to it. And, the implant gets its power wirelessly from the VPU. All of this implant is placed under the skull. That means that you cannot tell by looking at someone with the implant that they have it.

By the way, there is a predecessor device to the Orion called the Argus II.[3] However, unlike the Orion, it is implanted into the eye's retina. Therefore, it relies on the existing proper functioning of the eye and the optic nerves that connect the eyes with the brain. This means that the Argus II has a limited potential use. On the other hand, the Orion completely bypasses all of the structures of the eye including the optic nerves and directly stimulates the brain. As such, the Orion can be used regardless of the cause of blindness be it from an injury, glaucoma, macular degeneration or whatever.

For reasons too technical to get into here, it is thought that the Orion may be significantly more powerful than the Argus II. In the last chapter of this book, there is some background about much earlier work done regarding bionic vision. Although that earlier work is vastly less advanced and far less useful than is the Argus II let alone the Orion, work on bionic vision has in fact been ongoing for many decades.

Well, now that I had a basic understanding about the clinical trial and the

---

[3] Mark Humayunis is a professor of ophthalmology and biomedical engineering at the University of Southern California (USC). He spent 25 years creating the Argus. It is also made by Second Sight. It has been available since 2013. The Orion uses a significant amount of the same technology as does the Argus.

Orion, I now had to see if I could get into it. I knew this would not be easy. And, of course I had some fear about the whole thing. After all, it was a first-ever human experiment involving brain surgery. But, my fear of missing out on this was greater than my fear of all that. I simply had to try at least to get into the clinical trial!

Getting Into the Clinical Trial

My initial consultation at UCLA to see about getting into the Orion clinical trial was in early March, 2018. My wife, Charina, took me. As we waited in the lobby at the Department of Neurology, she whispered to me that there was a blind person already waiting ahead of me. "Surely, this person was there about the trial too," I worried. "Shoot," I thought! "Had I already missed the boat?" Indeed, I learned later that this person was there for the Orion trial.

After a little while, Sara Rodriguez greeted me. After filling-out the customary paperwork, we began to chat. I casually asked her, "So, how many calls have you had about the trial?"

Sara answered, "Oh, several hundred."

Again I thought to myself in horror "My God, I'm going to miss my chance!" So began my comradeship with Sara.

Then, I met with Dr. Nader Pouratian.[4] He is the neurosurgeon running the Orion trial

_____

[4] To learn more about Dr. Nader Pouratian, see the Acknowledgments section.

at UCLA. Of course, he is a world-class doctor. But, aside from all that, I must add that he is intelligent beyond description. I will mention some more about this in the chapter about getting the brain implant surgery later in this book. Suffice it to say that in this first meeting we each had several questions for one another. The bottom-line was that he thought that I might qualify for the trial, and I thought that I might want to do it. We would have many more meetings as time passed.[5]

The main thing that Dr. Pouratian stressed in this initial consultation was the experimental nature of the Orion trial. This had never been done before. And, it involves some risk. In the vast majority of clinical trials, taking some sort of a new drug is involved. This trial involves brain implant surgery to see if bionic vision might result. So, it would be riskier than a typical clinical trial.

Dr. Pouratian also explained to me the rudimentary, synthetic sort of vision that may be expected. In fact, there was no guarantee that it would work at all. I almost felt like he was trying to talk me out of doing it. But, no, he was simply laying it out for me in a matter-of-fact, scientific fashion. I had my reasons for wanting to do this. In the first chapter of this book, I mention some of the reasons why I did it.

---

[5] About a month after this first meeting, I had a meeting with Dr. Pouratian to address a number of questions I had before making my final decision. See Appendix A for what those questions were.

Later that same day of my initial consultation, I met with Soroush Niketeghad. He is one of the scientists at UCLA involved in the Orion trial. The purpose of our meeting was for me to have a chance to ask some questions about the trial. I would also be administered a "baseline" vision test. I will describe this baseline test in a subsequent chapter about the bionic laboratory. At some point in our meeting, Soroush asked me if I would like to see (really, hold and touch) the device. He meant the Orion's external hardware: the video processing unit, the glasses with the camera and the head strap. Later, I would see the implant itself. Of course, I said yes.

I put on the glasses, held the video processing unit in my hand and strapped-on the headband connecting the antenna to it. "WOW," I shouted out! Of course, it was not actually working. But, just to wear such a spectacular thing was amazing. I marveled at the technology that must surely be involved. Turning to Soroush I asked, "How much does this cost?"

Soroush chuckled at my ridiculous question. He rightly answered, "Richie, billions. There have been decades of scientific and medical advancements that have gone into the Orion. Anyway, it is not for sale at any price presently." I longingly wondered to myself if I would ever be so fortunate to have one of my very own. So ended my initial consultation at UCLA.

A few days after my initial consultation, Sara called me to say that we would proceed with the qualification process. I was thrilled! What I did not know then was that the qualification process involved numerous meetings with other doctors for them to judge my suitability for the trial. Over the next couple of months, there were meetings with a neural ophthalmologist, a psychiatrist, MRI brain scans, blood tests and on and on. I had been on many complex, stressful and multi-part job interviews in my life, but nothing compared to this! Honestly, all along the way I was pretty sure that something would come-up that would disqualify me.

Incidentally, at one meeting at UCLA to answer some questions I had about the trial and before being qualified, I was asked if I wanted to see (really hold and touch, of course) the brain implant itself. To be honest, I considered saying "No thanks" because it kind of freaked me out. But, instead I said "OK!" So, they dropped the implant into my hands. Then, they began to describe it to me. A little above, I describe the brain implant. You may have noticed yourself that it is not a small thing. Actually, it is sort of big. The cover of this book shows an x-ray of it in my head.

When most people think of a brain implant, they imagine some sort of a tiny microchip. Indeed, that is what I imagined before I actually held the real thing. Holding the implant in my hands, I wondered how this thing could even fit inside my head. The fear I had about putting this thing inside of my head was the closest I came to deciding not to be a participant in the Orion trial. Obviously, I got over it.

All along the way of this qualification process, I would periodically ask Sara how many participants had been accepted into the trial. Not more than five was the limit. As time progressed, she would give me the count: "one", "two", "three." Towards the end of my qualification process, the count was "four." At this point, I was so fearful that I might miss-out. "After going through all this," I would sometimes dreadfully think to myself!

Sara is my hero. Without giving me any special consideration, she in her methodical, professional style kept me moving well and good through the process. May 1, 2018, was among the greatest days in my life. On that day, Sara called me to say that I had been accepted. I would be the last participant accepted. "Five!"[6]

---

[6] Again, later a sixth participant was added. That sixth participant was added so that for reasons of efficiency and scale there would be a total of two participants at Baylor. Therefore, in the end there were four and two participants at UCLA and Baylor, respectively. However, at the time I was accepted into the trial I was the fifth, and final participant.

This Page Intentionally Left Blank

Chapter 3 - Brain Surgery to Implant Bionic Vision

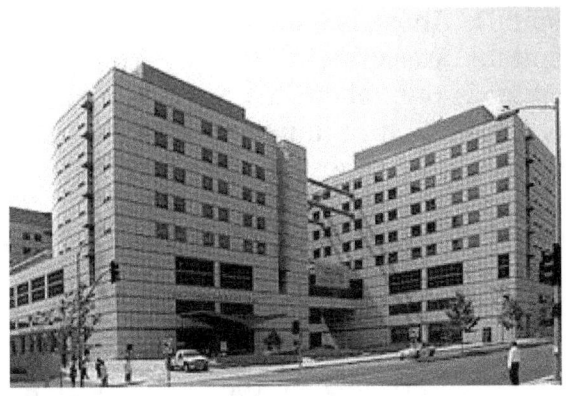

When I awoke on Thursday May 31, 2018, to go get my brain implant I was absolutely gripped by fear. Between that moment and when I would go under for the brain implant later that afternoon, there would be around 50 individual steps to take (e.g., get out of bed, walk to the bathroom, take a shower, ..., check-in at the hospital, get into the hospital gown, etc.). I said to my wife, Charina, "Sweetheart, there are like 50 steps I must take before I go under, and the only way I can do this is to take each step like a machine, one at a time." I progressed through each step robotically.

Now, it is one thing to get brain surgery when you *must*, like if you have had an injury or you have brain cancer. Let me assure you that it is an entirely different thing to do so *voluntarily*, when there is nothing wrong with you. This is especially true when the brain surgery is for the first-ever experimental implant for bionic vision.

The operation would take place at Ronald Reagan UCLA Medical Center (Ronald Regan Hospital). Above is a picture of Ronald Reagan Hospital. I was grateful for this. Ronald Regan Hospital is only about a 15-minute drive from where I live. More importantly, it is ranked as the seventh-best hospital in the US. It was completed in 2008 at a cost of over $1 billion. The Ronald Regan Hospital is considered to be the most technically advanced hospital in the US. If nothing else I knew I would be in good hands, I thought![7]

After arriving at the hospital at about 9:00 AM and checking-in, I had to sit around for a couple of hours. The operation was not scheduled until noon. The waiting around was interminable. Hearing numerous other patients checking-in for their necessary surgeries to treat a real medical problem did not help my nerves. Fear grew in me like a tea kettle on the stove getting ready to blow. "OK, just relax and go through one more step," I thought to myself.

While waiting in a small sitting room, a woman decided that she wanted to chat me up. Not only was I in no mood for a friendly chit-chat, but I wondered what I would say to her

---

[7] See the Wikipedia article about the Ronald Reagan Hospital here
https://en.wikipedia.org/wiki/Ronald_Reagan_UCLA_Medical_Center

when she inevitably would ask me, "So, what are you here for?"

"Well, I am here for an experimental first-ever brain implant for bionic vision," would have been my answer. Of course, she could see that I am blind. Really, I just wanted to be left alone to focus on remaining calm.

I was certain that her response after mulling it over in her mind for a moment would have been, "Yeah right! No, really, why are you here?" I did not want to go through all that. Mercifully, my wife Charina saw all this brewing and asked me if I would like to sit outside in the hallway. We did.

Going Under

At long last, I heard my name being called. I was led-off to a small pre-op ready room. There, I was instructed to get into the hospital gown. The anesthesiologist would come in soon, I was told. I have no shame in saying that it was at this point that I began to cry openly in fear. I thought about running out of the hospital. I felt like a trapped animal, like how a cat reacts when you try to take it to the vet. Even now, as I write these very words, I am crying a little bit remembering how scared I was. I could even hear my wife, Charina, crying a little too. But, she reached out and held my hand saying all would be fine. So I thought to myself, "OK Richie, go just one more step. Soon enough it will be too late to run away because you'll be put under."

Shortly, not one but *two* anesthesiologists came into the pre-op room. Then, some really smart woman came into the room too. I do not remember her name, but she explained to me that she was a brain surgeon and that she would be in the operating room together with Dr. Pouratian. I did not speak with Dr. Pouratian before going under. But, I found out that there would be like 10 people in the operating room - several brain surgeons, a couple of anesthesiologists, scientists from Second Sight, a crew of super nurses and a few others I am sure. I felt just a bit better because I thought to myself, "WOW! With all these sorts of people watching over me I would probably be OK."

Incidentally, I learned months after the operation that among the reasons the scientists from Second Sight are present during the operation is to make sure the Orion implant is working perfectly. They actually run a series of diagnostic tests on the implant to ensure that it is working perfectly before the doctors closed me all up. I am sure that the Second Sight scientists had a few back-ups with them, just in case. That's pretty smart! It had not occurred to me what a major bummer it would be to find out sometime later that the implant that was put into me was a dud!

One last thing I must say here. I begged the anesthesiologists to put me under *before* I was wheeled into the operating room. Through my tears of fear, I explained to them that it is terrible to lay in the operating room totally awake while all around you hearing surgical instruments clanking away and a bunch of random banter. As I mention in the Introduction to this book, I have had more than 50 operations before this one. So, I know that dreadfulness all too well. Those anesthesiologists were so wonderful! The last thing I remember before actually coming-to after the operation was my bed starting to move and the anesthesiologist saying to each other "So, how about those Dodgers!" They hit me with the drip before I got into the infernal operating room!

The first thing I heard after coming-to following the operation was Dr. Pouratian saying to me in a smiling voice from the foot of my bed, "Richie, you have a beautiful brain!" My first thought was to reply jokingly that I bet he says that to all the pretty girls. I did not say that. But, I was so happy to have a full understanding that I could still think clearly, that I still had my sense of humor and that I was not a vegetable.

Instead, I gave him a thumbs-up and replied, "OK, let's get to work!"

He responded, "Rest-up, and we'll see you soon!"

Going under deep, general anesthesia is truly bizarre. It really is like going into a time warp. It seemed to me like zero time had passed between the last thing I heard before going under "So, how about those Dodgers?" and the next thing I heard "Richie, you have a beautiful brain!" A moment later after Dr. Pouratian said those wonderful words, Charina was holding my hand. I knew then that I was OK.

After a while in the post-op recovery room, I was moved into a private room at the hospital. In fact, I understand that at Ronald Reagan Hospital all the rooms are private. My room was on the fourth floor. I think this is where all the brain surgery patients are. This was around 6:00 PM. I was not in any significant pain. That would change, as I explain later in this chapter. But, I felt pretty good. In fact, I was hungry and really thirsty. Charina and I had dinner together there in my private room.

A little later that night, say around 8:00 PM, I began to have some significant pain. Oddly, the pain was not coming from my head. Actually, my head itself really never had much pain. Instead, the pain was mostly in my neck. This is because of the position that the head is held in during brain surgery. I was warned about this by one of the anesthesiologists in the pre-op room before going under. He warned me that I would have a great amount of pain in my neck following the surgery. He said that it would last for about three weeks. In the pre-op room was the first time I heard about this. In hindsight, I am glad it went that way because I never had a chance to stress over it leading up to the operation. And, I sure am glad the anesthesiologist told me about it so that after the operation I was not surprised by this pain.

Anyway, I took a modest pain pill. A couple of hours later, I fell asleep. Around 10:00 PM, Charina went home to sleep. Everything seemed ordinary as my first night in the hospital following brain implant surgery settled-down.

Little did I know that I would soon have a spooky visitor in the dead of the night.

A Spooky Visitor in the Dead of the Night

Before I tell you about this strange happening, let me say a few things first. I am not necessarily saying here that anything conspiratorial, mystical or religious happened. And, this was not a dream or some sort of a drug-induced hallucination either. But, it did happen. Also, I do not believe that anything untoward, inappropriate or troublesome occurred. Whatever this was, I am sure that there is some logical, normal and rational explanation for it.

I awoke at what I thought was very late in the evening the same day as the surgery (Thursday), but later learned that it was actually around 2:00 AM the following morning (Friday). A spooky feeling crept over me that I was being watched. After a moment, indeed I heard a voice at the foot of my bed say very calmly, "Hey pal. How are you feeling?" He sounded just like the character Gordon Gekko (played by Michael Douglas) from the 1987 movie <u>Wall Street</u>. For some unknown reason, I felt no fear but, rather, strangely comforted that I was being watched over.

The visitor seemed to be in his 50s. As I imagined in my mind how he might look, he seemed to look like Gordon Gekko besides just sounding like him! He then asked me a few more questions about how I was feeling and did a few neurological and cognitive tests. Basically, these cognitive tests were things like counting on my fingers, pulling on his hands with both of mine, asking me if I knew where I was and what the date was and so on. To his pleasure, and mine too, all these tests I performed perfectly. At this point, I assumed that the visitor was merely a doctor whom I had not yet met.

He then asked if I were in any pain. I told him that about eight hours earlier I was given a modest pain pill, but that at that moment I was only in a slight amount of pain. The pain was mostly in my neck. I was, however, entirely sober and clear minded as we chatted. The pain pill had completely worn off by then. He then seemed to look around to ensure that no one was watching, and in an apparent desire not to offend Big Pharma said to me, "You know, you'd be better off just taking Tylenol instead of narcotics because Tylenol promotes healing." "Would you like me to order you some," he asked?

I said, "Sure." He then walked to one end of my room, and I could hear him typing away on the computer.

We chatted a bit more. After a little while he then said, "OK pal, we'll see you soon." He patted my leg, and then left the room. About a half an hour later, a nurse came into my room and gave me a couple of Tylenol pills. I fell back asleep.

Now here's where it gets weird. Later in the morning that same day (Friday) the Charge Nurse, whom I had met the previous evening around 10:00 PM as she started her shift came into my room. She said that it was 7:00 AM, that she was finishing her shift, asked how I was feeling and if I needed any pain pills. I told her that I did not need any pain pills because the Tylenol pills the doctor from much earlier in the morning got for me were working great.

The Charge Nurse said with some amount of confusion, "What doctor? What Tylenol?" I told her all about the visitor I had much earlier that morning. She said with some amount of concern, "Richie, I have been on duty since 10:00 PM last night. There has been no doctor on this floor let alone any doctor seeing you."

She then went to the end of my room where the computer was. I heard her typing away on it. After a bit of clicking away on the computer, she said, "Well, yes indeed at around 2:00 AM this morning Tylenol was ordered for you." Then, she said with an increased level of concern, "Huh, the screen for which doctor ordered that Tylenol is blank. Let me look into just what went-on."

Not wanting to blow anyone's cover, I said to her, "No, that's OK, let's just let it be. Everything is fine."

Reluctantly, she said, "OK" and excused herself. I never saw this particular Charge Nurse again. Nor did I ever find out just who this spooky visitor in the dead of the night was. To the spooky visitor, I hope to meet you again someday!

Incidentally, what the spooky visitor said about Tylenol promoting healing turned-out to be very true. Taking Tylenol then became a regular thing for me. About a month after the surgery, everyone was amazed at how nicely my surgical scar was healing. About ten months after the surgery, they said that if they did not know I had had brain surgery they couldn't tell by looking at my head. The picture on the left (below) shows my head just a few days after the operation. The picture on the right (below) shows my head about ten months later. At most,

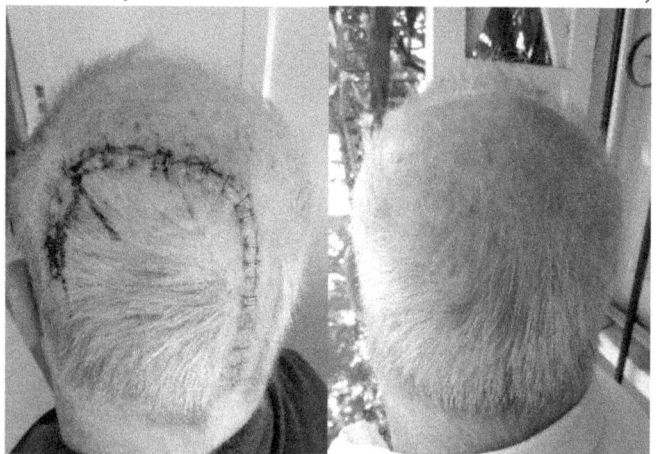

people said it looks like maybe a cat scratched my head.

Only Three Days Later I Went Home

Oddly, I never had much pain at all in my head itself. That surprised me. You would think that a brain implant might result in a great amount of pain in your head. But, no. In fact, were it not for the neck pain I suffered, I might not have needed any pain pills at all. Well, perhaps some Tylenol.

The rest of that day Friday and all the day Saturday I steadily grew stronger. Sunday, I went home. However, all the while that damnable neck pain was excruciating. Indeed, to deal with it I would need heavy pain pills for about the next four days. After that, just good-old Tylenol! It was just as the anesthesiologist said, the neck pain would last for three weeks following the surgery.

Let me say just a few words about a couple of neat things that happened at Ronald Reagan Hospital during my stay there. Wonderfully, the food was fantastic. Hospital food is notorious for how bad it is. Nothing could be further from the truth at Ronald Reagan Hospital. It is like being in a five-star hotel. Really, you have a full menu from which you order whatever you want, whenever you want it and however much of it you might like. I ate like a king. My huge appetite probably was a result of my body craving nutrients for healing. All that good eating likely contributed to my fast recovery too!

I am saving the best for last - the super and adorable nurses. They were so competent that they make other nursing staff look sophomoric. Aside from that, they were so nice to me. They would come into my room all the time, even at the wee hours of the night as I had my usual insomnia, just to chat me up. On more than one occasion, those wonderful nurses would go foraging in the small hours of the night (like 2:00 AM or 3:00 AM) for my favorite flavored popsicle stick (grape). Sometimes, they could not find my favorite flavor on my own floor. Undeterred, they would search the hospital high and low for it. One night, a wonderful nurse searched three different floors to find my favorite flavor! Before my brain implant operation, I only liked popsicle sticks so-so. Now, I absolutely love them!

Most adorably, apparently the rumor had spread among the nurses that I had had experimental brain implant surgery for bionic vision. Seemingly, the gossip left-out the nature of the Orion - not the least of which is that the implant is only half of the system. That is, you need to wear the external hardware (e.g., the glasses with the camera, the video processing unit) to transmits the video stream to the brain implant. This fact mattered not at all to them. The nurses often came into my room saying to me girlishly, "Richie, can you see me now?" Sometimes I would walk the halls together with my wife, Charina. I could feel the nurses gazing at me in bewilderment. With great expectation, they fully expected that at any moment I would suddenly see them in full glory. I suspect that, there, these nurses regularly see miracles. So, for them, it is not so hard to believe in bionic vision.

To sum it up, I went home Sunday - three days after brain implant surgery. A week after the surgery, Charina and I would be walking around our neighborhood. We were in amazement that only a week earlier I had brain surgery. A month after the surgery, it was time to get to work learning how to see again in a

whole new way. So, off to the bionic laboratory
I went!

This Page Intentionally Left Blank

Chapter 4 - The Bionic Laboratory

A month after the brain implant surgery, I began going to the bionic laboratory at UCLA about once a week. Each visit would be for about three hours. This was in July of 2018. There, I began to work with some of the most remarkable people I have ever met: the scientists from Second Sight, the maker of the Orion. And, besides the technology of the Orion itself discussed in the previous chapter, the technology employed at the bionic lab is out of this world. The great science fiction writer Arthur C. Clarke once wrote "Any sufficiently advanced technology is indistinguishable from magic." Of course, Arthur C. Clarke is the writer of the movie 2001: A Space Odyssey (1968) directed by Stanley Kubrick.

Believe me, Arthur would think that this is all magic. As you will read below, it becomes difficult to distinguish between technology and magic. Later in this chapter, I will talk about exactly what I began to see and just what happens in the bionic lab. But first, let me say a little more about the technology of the Orion and the Second Sight scientists.

The technology of the Orion can only be described as other worldly. In the previous chapter, I described how it came about under the FDA's "Break-through Device Program." The purpose of that Program is to pull-forward technologies that are way out on the cutting-edge of science and technology and which have

37

a reasonable chance of addressing severe medical conditions. The Orion's technology is, I would guess, about 20 years or more beyond what might have been otherwise available. In fact, the Defense Advanced Research Projects Agency (DARPA) makes no secret about its funding and promotion of these types of technologies. DARPA even openly discusses its decades-long work in this area on its own website. Indeed, DARPA has had a hand in developing technologies very similar to the Orion.[8] You may be interested in a bit more reading about DARPA's publicly announced, ongoing work in further advancing these technologies in the last chapter of this book regarding the future of bionic vision.

The primary Second Sight scientists with whom I work in the bionic lab were Uday Patel and Michelle Armenta Salas.[9] Another Senior Research Scientist from Second Sight, Vara Wuyyuru, would also come to the bionic lab from time-to-time. I will talk a bit more about Uday below, and about Vara in the next chapter. But, let me relay a little story about the first time I met Michelle. This illustrates the sort of people these Second Sight scientists are.

On my first day in the bionic lab, I met Michelle. She is a young woman. I asked her to tell me a little about herself. She began to say in

---

[8] As a small example of how far out DARPA is, it invented the Internet, stealth technology, GPS and self-driving car technology to name a few.
[9] See the Acknowledgements section for more about Uday and Michelle.

the most humdrum, no big deal voice "Well, Richie, I got my Ph.D. from Arizona State University in brain-machine interfacing. [10] Then, I did some postdoctoral work at Cal-Tech with paraplegic individuals with brain implants to control movement of a robotic hand only with their thoughts. My specialty is helping people train their brains to work with brain implants. Now, I am working with Second Sight to help you."

"What," I exclaimed! "Back the truck up one moment, Michelle! They already have Ph.D. programs in brain-machine interfacing," I asked her?

"Yeah," Michele replied as if this were an everyday, no big deal sort of thing.

Honestly, I must say that all of these people involved in the Orion are super-human. That there are people who are so smart and who devote their entire lifetime to something so far out as this is an incredible thing. People like Uday, Michelle and all their kind are right up there, if not beyond, the scientists who got us to the moon. The brain power brought to bear on the Orion is beyond comprehension.

What I See with Bionic Vision

Perhaps a better description than "bionic vision" would be "synthetic vision." That is, what I see is nothing like what normally sighted people see. It is not color or even black-and-

---

[10] Often, "brain-machine interfacing" is also called "brain-computer interfacing" or BCI.

white. It is not even grey-scale. It is a bit more like monochrome. And, there is no sharp definition either. Instead, things are more like orbs or blobs of light.

Another thing is that what I see is all in my mind's eye. That is, it is all in my head. If you close your eyes and then imagine the international symbol for the Red Cross, you are seeing a thick red cross in your mind's eye. If I imagine this same symbol, I see in my mind's eye the same thing as you do. Another way to think about this is to consider what you see when you dream. When you dream, it is all in your mind's eye. In the last chapter of this book about the future of bionic vision, there will be a bit more to say about what is seen when dreaming.

As a matter of fact, all vision - even for sighted people - happens in the mind's eye; that is, in the brain. The physical structures of the eye itself including the optic nerve are merely a pipeline to get an electrical impulse to the brain.[11] One of the many wonders of the Orion is that it bypasses those physical structures and sends electrical impulses straight to the brain. This makes the Orion a potential solution for blind people everywhere regardless of the cause

---

[11] The brain seems not to care a whole lot about *how* it gets electrical signals but, rather, that it just gets them in a consistent way. This subject relates to something known as "neural plasticity. In the next chapter, it will be further described. And, there is a reference to an incredible video link (a TED Talk) on this topic in that chapter too.

of their blindness, be it from glaucoma, retinal damage, physical injury or whatever.

Now, imagine an old-school air traffic controller's radar scope from the 1960s. That is what I see in my mind's eye with the Orion. Objects that are within the field of view of the camera in the Orion's eyeglasses flash in my mind's eye. In the next chapter, I will talk a bit more about the nature of this synthetic, bionic vision. I will also describe the factors that drive the quality of this vision, and how that quality changes. But, for now, simply imagine you have a radar scope in your mind's eye.

The Bionic Lab

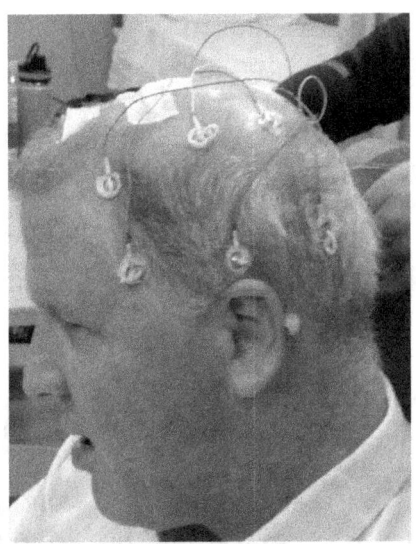

My first visit to the bionic lab happened in July 2018. It is at UCLA. I typically go there once a week for about three hours each visit. Primarily, I work with the Second Sight scientists, Uday and Michelle. The work at the bionic lab is, essentially, broken-up into two phases. The first phase is all about ensuring that the Orion is safe. The picture above shows me in the lab wired-up with 23 electrodes on my head to monitor my brain waves.[12] That phase lasted until mid-September 2018. The second phase then began. This second phase is mostly about tinkering with the Orion. This tinkering involves improving *what* I see with it, and also learning *how* to see with it.

In the first phase at the bionic lab, I was hooked-up to 23 brainwave electrodes to monitor the functioning of my brain (pictured above), had an IV in me, had my vital signs monitored and laid in a bed. There were typically at least four people in the room with me at all times: the scientists from Second Sight Uday and Michelle, the brainwave technician and a UCLA graduate student (often Soroush Niketeghad). There were always nurses just outside my door too. Besides the brainwave technician there in the room monitoring me, that monitoring was streamed across the campus at UCLA where a doctor at the Department of Neurology kept an eye on it. The IV was in me just in case I had any trouble. I never did.

I must say here how wonderful Sara Rodriguez was. She would be in the bionic lab

---

[12] This is called Electroencephalography or EEG. It is used for monitoring electrical activity of the brain. See this Wikipedia article for more:
https://en.wikipedia.org/wiki/Electroencephalography

for the beginning of every visit. I really do not like needles. At every visit to the bionic lab during this first phase, Sara held my hand for the IV needle stick. Often people would say to me, "Richie, you volunteered for experimental brain implant surgery! How could you possibly be afraid of a little needle prick?" Well, this cannot be explained. Suffice it to say that I am terrified of needles. Sara made it all OK for me. The power of compassion and the human touch is grossly understated. Sara has my unending gratitude and respect. She is exemplary of the outstanding sorts of people who work at UCLA.

Prior to my first visit to the bionic lab, I asked Uday if it was like the bionic lab in The Six Million Dollar Man?[13] That is, I asked him if the lab had computers the size of refrigerators with reel-to-reel tapes, scientists in white lab coats with clipboards and pocket protectors scampering all around, lots of monitors, doctors and nurses and so on. Uday chuckled a little and answered, "Well, Richie, everything you mentioned is true except for the computers. Nowadays there are a couple of laptops." He was spot-on.

---

[13] The Six Million Dollar Man was a hit 1970s TV series about a NASA astronaut who becomes severely injured in a crash of an experimental aircraft. The astronaut is "rebuilt" in an operation that costs $6 million (more than $33 million in today's money). His right arm, both legs and the left eye are replaced with bionic implants that enhance his strength, speed and vision far above human norms. See this link: https://en.wikipedia.org/wiki/The_Six_Million_Dollar _Man

Uday and Michelle would always bring along with them to the bionic lab their laptops and other high-tech stuff. As you might have noticed from the foregoing, the technology at the bionic lab is out of this world. On my first day in the bionic lab I asked Uday, "Let me know when we crossover into the unknown realms of science and medical technology."

He answered "Richie, we are already there!"

So, this first phase in the bionic lab focused on calibrating the Orion and making sure that it was safe for me. Uday and Michelle would "ping" my brain implant by sending electrical impulses to it. This is done to determine the threshold levels necessary to cause a flash of light in my mind's eye. On the first day in the bionic lab when they sent the first ping, I nearly cried. I saw a little flash of light! It was the first time I had seen *anything* for 13 years. A lot of time was spent with them pinging me. I would also describe just *what* I saw and *where* in my mind's eye I saw it. This is called "mapping."

These threshold and mapping calibration exercises continue periodically to this day. As I will explain further in the next chapter regarding the factors that determine the quality of what I see, the process of continuously tinkering with the Orion is perpetual. The goal is always to improve what I see.

Now, this may not be anything special for sighted people, but one day in the bionic lab I saw a purple flash. Color! And, it was the most beautiful shade of purple - electric purple. It was SO pretty. I had not seen any colors for 13 years. However, this was an anomaly. I do not see colors. Nor am I likely to see colors anytime in my lifetime. Really, what I see is in monochrome. I will have a little more to say about color in the last chapter of this book about the future of bionic vision, though. Anyway, I saw purple. It was glorious!

In the second phase of the bionic lab, mercifully I would not be hooked-up to the IV. Nor am I connected to the 23 brainwave electrodes. In this second phase of the bionic lab, it is primarily about testing to determine just what I am able to see and also learning techniques to interpret what I do see. Of course, there is always diagnostic, threshold and mapping tinkering happening. Uday and Michelle are always monitoring and adjusting everything on their laptops.

One major thing we do in the bionic lab are a series of tests where I am looking at a 21-inch touch screen monitor. In the previous chapter, I referred to these tests as "baseline" tests. Most everyone has had an eye test where you read the smallest row of letters they can see on a chart. This chart is called a Snellen eye chart. The top row of this chart has just one letter, a big "E." If that is the best you can read, your vision is 20/200. "20/200" means that what a normally sighted person can see at 200 feet away you can see from 20 feet away. At 20/200, you are considered legally blind.

Now, if your eyesight is less than legally blind, but not totally blind, you basically are considered to be visually impaired or to have very low vision. This is the area where these baseline tests are used to assess eyesight. There are three basic baseline eye tests: the Square Localization, the Direction of Motion and the Grading Visual Acuity tests. You will recall from the previous chapter that I took these baseline tests on my initial consultation at UCLA before being accepted into the Orion trial. At that time, I failed them all miserably. However, early-on in phase two of the bionic lab, some remarkable things began to happen. I will describe some of these remarkable happenings in the following section.

Remarkable Happenings in the Bionic Lab

In early October 2018, one day at the bionic lab I took the Square Localization test, mentioned in the previous section. Basically, for this test, an approximate three-inch white square on a black background appears in various spots on the touch screen monitor. The objective is to touch the square. Remembering that the last time I took this test as a "baseline" at my initial consultation before being accepted into the trial, I scored zero. Well, this time, with the Orion, I basically scored 100%. That is, before the Orion I saw nothing. But, with the Orion, I could actually see something on the screen. And, I could reach out and touch it!

Believe me, everyone in the bionic lab was stunned - not the least of which was me. I can tell you that, for me at least, to be able to detect something - anything - on the screen was stunning. It nearly caused me to faint.

I did not expect this, and I do not think anyone else expected this either. Let me tell you that as I gazed at the screen with my bionic vision, I paused for long moments in sheer magical bewilderment that I could actually *see* something! Even today, and as I write these very words, my eyes tear-up and I get a little choked-up. This was among the most wonderful moments in my whole life.

About a week later in the bionic lab, I took the Direction of Motion and the Grading Visual Acuity tests. The Direction of Motion test, essentially, has a white bar about a half an inch thick and about three inches long on a black background. The bar moves across the touch screen in various directions (e.g., down, up, left, right, diagonally from all four corners of the screen, etc.). The objective here is to swipe with your finger on the touch screen in whatever direction you see the bar moving.

As for the Grading Visual Acuity test, basically, lines in various thicknesses and in various directions (horizontal, vertical, diagonal, etc.) appear on the touch screen. These lines alternate between black and white. They also progressively decrease in their thickness. As the thickness of the lines decreases, it becomes increasingly harder to see in what orientation they are. In this test, the objective is to say in which orientation you see the lines going.

For both the Grading Visual Acuity and the Direction of Motion test, you have increasingly less time to react and answer the particular objective. That is, the time to say in what orientation lines are and the speed at which the bar moves across the screen is getting shorter. These two tests, the Direction of Motion and the Grading Visual Acuity tests, are harder than the Square Localization test.

However, remembering that when I first took these two Direction of Motion and Grading Visual Acuity tests without the Orion, I scored zero, but now with the Orion when I took them again I scored about 50%. And, this was on my first try! About another week later in the bionic lab, I took these two tests once again. This time, I scored much better. That is a 50% improvement! There are several factors that drive the quality of what I see. These factors came into play here. They will be explored a bit further in the next chapter.

Chapter 5 - Coming Home with Bionic Vision

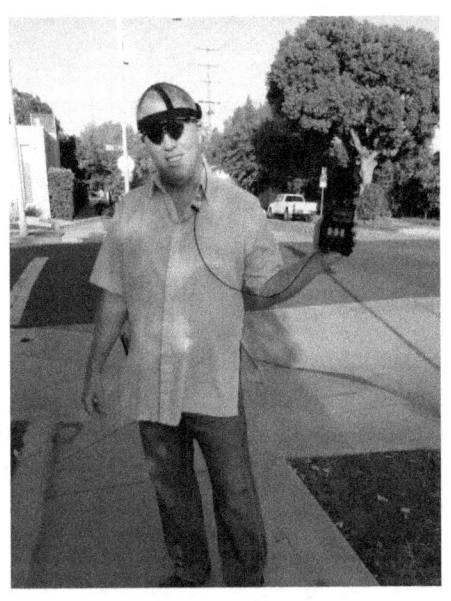

In late October 2018, I came home with the Orion (sometimes called "the device"). This is considered to have happened earlier than what was expected. The reason for this acceleration is that things were going very well. In a September 2018 press release, Second Sight said that "The Company recently completed enrollment of the first five [there are actually now six] subjects, ahead of schedule, with Orion as part of Second Sight's early feasibility clinical study. All five subjects have had their Orion systems activated, and all subjects reported seeing light from virtually all electrodes ... . As a result of these successes, the Company is now progressing with more complex testing ... ."[14] That same press release went on to say that, based on these early results, Second Sight anticipates starting an expanded study of the Orion in 2019.

So, things were going well not only for me but for everyone. Now, before I go further, I want to explain some more about just what I see. From the previous chapter, I explained that basically what I see is like a radar scope in my mind's eye. And, that "scope" is monochrome. What I see are pulsing lights that vary in their intensity based on whatever is within the field of view of the camera mounted in the device's glasses. For example, looking at a light that is turned on causes a bright pulsing light whereas looking at the TV would cause a slightly less bright pulsing light. None of this has much definition to it. Several factors that drive the quality of what is seen would, however, begin to come into play. These factors are described next.

The factors that determine the Quality of What is Seen

The main factors that determine how well someone sees with the device are the person's mental attitude, training with the

---

[14] See Second Sight's September 4, 2018, press release "Second Sight Appoints Pat Ryan Chief Operating Officer" at this link:
https://www.businesswire.com/news/home/201809040 05269/en/

device, neural plasticity and technological advancement of the device. One day in the bionic lab while working with Vara Wuyyuru, a Senior Research Scientist with Second Sight, she explained to me that she believes that the most important factor of them all is the first of these factors - a person's overall mental attitude. That is, how positive in life a person is, how much they *believe* in the device's ability to help them and their overall outlook on life in general is all-important. This is, of course, an unquantifiable and somewhat mysterious factor. Vara knows more than just a little bit about this. For more than 10 years, she has been working on these technologies and with people using the Orion and its predecessor device (the Argus II).

Something more must be said here about Vara's observations regarding the power of positive thinking and the power of belief. Personally, I found her observations fascinating. Vara, and all of her colleagues for that matter, are extremely educated, experienced and sophisticated scientists. Indeed, the same can be said about the doctors at UCLA. And yet, none of these people are shy at all about recognizing that there are mysterious and presently not well understood forces involved when dealing with the deep workings of the mind. Put another way, way out here on the outer limits of science, there may be things going on beyond the scope of how we understand things today. Personally, I find this open-mindedness very inspiring and exciting. These traits of the Second Sight scientists and the UCLA doctors are a supreme sign of very intelligent people. These are the people who will solve these mysteries.[15]

Training on how to see with the Orion's bionic, synthetic vision is really important. As with everything in life, training and practice improves how well you do. With the Orion, the vision that is produced by it is not at all like what normally sighted people see. So, there are specific techniques, tactics and tricks that can be used to help interpret what is seen.

Vara taught me a few simple techniques one day in the bionic lab when I took the Direction of Motion and the Grading Visual Acuity tests. A big reason why I did better on these tests the next time I took them (as mentioned above) is because of what Vara taught me. Over time, Vara would continue to teach me amazing things about how to see with the Orion. I simply cannot figure-out how she knows these things. What she does is like explaining to someone blind from birth the

---

[15] Now, neither I, Vara, her colleagues at Second Sight nor the doctors at UCLA are saying in all this that "God" or some mystical forces are involved here. On the other hand, and this is merely my opinion, I do not think that any of us are firmly ruling that out. Perhaps this really is nothing more than science. But, if so, it is science that is just not understood today. Is it not curious that if you were to ask a Professor of Astronomy how much is correct in a 500 year old astronomy textbook, they would reply that nearly all of it is incorrect based on what we understand today? As a child growing-up, in church there was a wise old priest named Monsignor John V. Sheridan who would often refer to such things as "the great mysteries of life." Indeed, Monsignor.

color blue. Think about that for a moment. How would you describe the color blue to someone blind from birth? Remember, you cannot use other colors in your explanation. In fact, you cannot use anything of a visual nature in your explanation. How accurately would the blind person understand the color blue after your explanation? Somehow, Vara can do this sort of thing.

Another aspect of training with the Orion is some specialized coaching I get for it. In early November 2018, I began working with what are called low vision rehabilitation specialists. However, *these* rehab specialists are not your everyday sort. Besides all the regular education, certification and training that regular low vision rehabilitation specialists have, these rehab specialists have specific training and experience working with people who have the Orion - like me.

Let me draw an analogy here. Suppose you just started to learn to play tennis. Well, if you began to train with a tennis pro you would learn how to play tennis much faster and much better than if you never trained with a tennis pro. Later in this chapter, I will talk some more about training with rehab specialists. For now, enough has been said just to understand that a great amount of training on how to see with the Orion was (and still is) undertaken.

The "X-Factor" in determining how well someone can see with the Orion is the concept of neural plasticity. Essentially, neural plasticity is the brain's uncanny ability to rewire itself to learn how to do something in a totally new way. As an example, it is commonly believed that the blind can hear much better than sighted people. Generally, this is true. Among the reasons for this is that brain power is diverted from other functions, like vision, to hearing thereby resulting in better hearing.[16] This is, technically, neural plasticity in action. This topic is a bit too complex to go into deeply here, but Wikipedia has a great article on it including material on neural plasticity as it relates to vision, human echo location and more.[17]

A much better way to explain neural plasticity is Stanford Professor Dr. David Eagleman's amazing TED Talk "Can we create new senses for humans"?[18] Basically, the brain seems not to care a whole lot about *how* it gets information but, instead, only that it gets it in a consistent way. If it does, somehow the brain begins to figure it out and will rewire itself as need be. As Dr. Eagleman explains in his TED Talk, human biological structures like the eye are merely "peripheral equipment" (like a keyboard) that convert information (like typing)

---

[16] See the blog post "Do the Brains of Blind Persons 'Rewire' or Adjust to Significantly Enhance the Other Senses? New Research Says Yes." at this link: https://www.visionaware.org/blog/visionaware-blog/do-the-brains-of-blind-persons-rewire-or-adjust-to-significantly-enhance-the-other-senses-new-research-says-yes/12

[17] See this link for the Wikipedia article on neural plasticity: https://en.wikipedia.org/wiki/Neuroplasticity

[18] See this link for Dr. Eagleman's video: https://www.ted.com/talks/david_eagleman_can_we_create_new_senses_for_humans?language=en

into an electrical signal which are sent to the brain (the computer). You really ought to watch this "Ted Talk." It will forever change how you perceive things.

As mentioned previously, all of our senses including vision are ultimately created in the brain. The eyes simply convert light into electrical signals which are carried over the optic nerve to the brain. Well, the Orion uses its camera to capture light which is then converted into electrical signals which are then transmitted straight to the brain. *Voila*! Ta-da! Presto! Simple, right?

The processes by which the brain accomplishes neural plasticity are not well understood. It is, however, well known that the brain does in fact do this. Also, although there seems to be a better ability for younger people to benefit from neural plasticity, even much older people retain a great ability for this. And, there seems to be a degree of variability among individuals in their neural plasticity capabilities, just in the same way that people have varying athletic or academic capabilities.

So, the degree to which neural plasticity will impact use of the Orion is unknown. It is the "X-Factor." For sure, there are many unknown things about how the Orion will work. Many, many things involved with it are beyond what is presently well understood.

The last factor that will impact how well someone can see with the Orion is its technological advancement. Right now, I am on what I call "version 1.0." One thing is for sure though, like all technology its advancement is likely to be rapid and dramatic. As an example, 12 years ago version 1 of the iPhone was introduced. Now, we are on version 10 (Apple calls it roman numeral "X"). The difference between the technology in the iPhone 1 versus the iPhone 10 is dazzling. I will say quite a bit more about this in the last chapter of this book regarding the future of bionic vision.

Training with Rehab Specialists

Learning to see with synthetic vision is not easy, to say the least. Earlier, I explained what I see and how different this vision is as compared to how normally sighted people see. But, there is much more that makes it different and hard to learn. For one thing, I have no depth perception. My world is two dimensional: up and down, and left and right. There is no near and far. However, I do get other information about my surroundings. For example, of course what I hear gives me clues about the distance of things. In the next chapter, I will talk more about some of the differences and challenges of synthetic vision and how I have adapted to them. No doubt, working with highly trained low vision rehab specialists to learn how to see with the Orion helps me develop these adaptations.

An odd and somewhat unexpected thing for me about beginning to use the Orion is how exhausting it is. Although this was a surprise to me, it was not a surprise to the Second Sight scientists. They told me this would happen. In my early stages of using it, I would become very weary after using it for only an hour or two. This is true both in the bionic lab and when I first came home with it. Now, this is not a physical type of exhaustion but, instead, a mental exhaustion. If you have ever been in really difficult classes in school (like math, chemistry or physics) or attended training at your workplace where they cram-in tons of information, then you know this sort of mental exhaustion. Over time, though, my endurance would increase.

Undoubtedly, this mental exhaustion is a result of neural plasticity (discussed above) working away. I can *feel* my brain exercising. If you have ever noticed when you begin to use your computer, as you increasingly multitask (watching YouTube, checking your email, making a post on Facebook, sending out a Tweet, etc.), you can hear the cooling fans stepping-up their speed. Your computer is working increasingly harder and harder. It is heating-up. I think this is similar to what is happening in my brain due to the workings of neural plasticity. Unlike a computer, though, I just get tired. After using the Orion for any significant period of time, I just want to take a nap.

Curiously, I learned from a rehab specialist that this mental exhaustion is not only normal but a good thing. It turns-out that the magic of neural plasticity happens mostly while we sleep. Much the same way as when learning a musical instrument, it is best done in small increments like 15 minutes at a time. Then, taking a break is recommended. This is opposed to long sessions like hours on end without taking a break. The same is true for learning to see with the Orion. Working in small doses and then napping allows the brain to rewire itself.

Working with the rehab specialists really caused my brain to work hard! I first met with Mickey Damelio in mid-November 2018. He is a Senior Vision Rehabilitation Manager at Second Sight.[19] We met in the bionic lab at UCLA. In this first meeting, we did a few fantastic exercises. They are described next.

Mickey laid-out on the table in front of me a black cloth that is about three feet wide and two feet long. The first test was placing a white cloth that is about 4 inches square randomly on the black cloth. My task was to find it. I did it pretty well! My hand-eye coordination(sort-to-speak) was a little off a couple of times, but mostly I was dead-on. If you are interested, about a week earlier my wife took a video of me at home doing a "find the plate" task which I invite you to see for yourself.[20] It was a little easier than the find the cloth test that Mickey conducted here.

The next test we did was to lay-out three different squares randomly on the table in front

---

[19] Mickey's education, experience and accomplishments within the area of low vision rehabilitation are very impressive. See Mickey's LinkedIn webpage here: https://www.linkedin.com/in/mickey-damelio-b5034b155

[20] To see the video of the "find the plate" test, go to this link: https://www.dropbox.com/s/dmpni23218ndq7v/find_the_plate.mp4?raw=1

of me. Each cloth was about four inches square. However, this time one cloth was solid white, one cloth was a black-and-white checker pattern with small squares and one cloth was a black-and-white checker pattern with large squares. My task was first to find each cloth, and then to place them in a row from left to right with the solid cloth first, the small checker pattern next and the large checker pattern last. Finding each of the three cloths was pretty easy. But arranging them in proper order was something different.

As I gazed at each cloth in front of me with my bionic eye, I thought a bit about how things appear on a radar scope. Remember, a close analogy to what my bionic, synthetic vision looks like is similar to a monochrome radar scope. I reasoned that the cloth with the strongest, brightest flashing of light in my mind's eye must be the solid cloth. Of the three, it should have the greatest contrast and thus response. Likewise, the next strongest response in my mind's eye ought to be the cloth with the small checker pattern since it has more contrast than the cloth with the large checker pattern, but less than the solid cloth. This would leave the cloth with the large checker pattern. In theory, that cloth should have the weakest response of the three.

Using this theory, I lined them up. Lo and behold, I did it correctly! Everyone in the bionic lab was stunned, especially me. This way of interpreting how patterns appear to me plays a huge role in seeing with synthetic vision. In the next chapter, I will explain this a little further by way of how skilled radar operators do their job where I talk about getting to know my bionic vision.

The third test Mickey gave me was really remarkable. He put a small white ball in my hand. This ball is about the size of a pea. It is made out of a foam rubber material. Mickey then told me that he would randomly place five of these little white balls on the table in front of me. My task would be to find each one and remove it from the table.

I had a little trouble finding the first one. But, Mickey and the Second Sight scientists that were also present said it was a bit unfair because there was some reflection on the table surrounding that particular ball. The next three balls I got pretty easily. My hand-eye coordination was off just a little bit. Frankly, I could hardly believe that I could detect these little white balls at all, let alone their location on the table in front of me.

The stunning thing was when I went for the fifth and final ball. I reached out and placed my fingers down on the table around where I thought I saw the ball. My fingers formed a circle about the size of a can of Coke. I did not feel anything. I then sadly announced that somehow I must have missed it. After a brief moment, one of the Second Sight scientists, Uday, said "No, Richie. Close your fingers." I closed my fingers. Bullseye! My fingers were surrounding this last little white ball. I nailed it!

And so concluded my first day working with Mickey. There would be many more days working with him to come. My way forward learning to see with bionic, synthetic vision would be hard and long. There would be many frustrating moments, but there would also be many glorious victories.

This Page Intentionally Left Blank

Chapter 6 – Learning to See with Bionic Vision

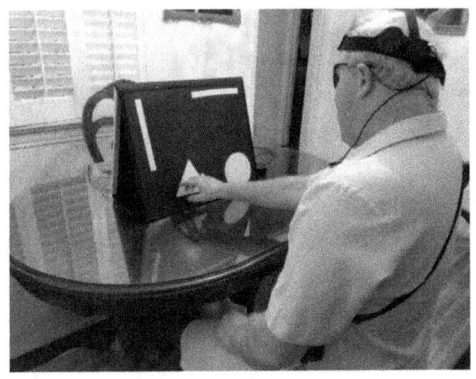

One day at the bionic lab, I met Dr. Greenberg.[21] Although it cannot be, if any single person could be credited with the invention of the Orion, it would be him. He expressed to me that, at times, progress learning to see with bionic vision would seem slow. Dr. Greenberg told me that sometimes I would become frustrated. He also said that, over time, I would

[21] Robert J. Greenberg, M.D., Ph.D. is a co-founder of Second Sight. He previously served as Second Sight's Chairman, President and CEO. For over a decade, Dr. Greenberg has been the Chairman of the Alfred Mann Foundation, where he now is its Executive Chairman. Dr. Greenberg is credited with countless patents in the medical devices Field. He has been inducted as a National Academy of Inventors Fellow. In the late 1990s, Dr. Greenberg served as lead reviewer at the Office of Device Evaluation at the FDA in the Neurological Devices Division. Dr. Greenberg has been working on bionic vision for 30 years.

be amazed with what I could see. On a day-to-day basis, progress would seem imperceptible. But, when measured by the years, it would be remarkable. Dr. Greenberg pointed out to me that, after all, my visual cortex had been asleep for 13 years! In scope and scale, meeting Dr. Greenberg felt like meeting Thomas Edison, Bill Gates or Steven Jobs.

In the previous chapter, I discussed the concept of neural plasticity. Since the part of my brain responsible for vision (the visual cortex) had been asleep for 13 years, it would require vigorous exercise and training to get back into shape. Put another way, if you were paralyzed in bed for 13 years and then suddenly had the ability to walk, it would not be something that you could simply jump up and do. Slow, steady baby steps would be required. For me, slow, steady rehabilitation of my visual cortex would be required. To learn to see with bionic vision, I would need to exercise my brain like how an Olympic gymnast trains with the uneven bars.

And so, at the end of November 2018 I began my rehab training. First, I began learning to walk around my neighborhood. With the Orion, I could detect the sidewalk and distinguish it from other things in front of me. I also used my cane. This was the most independent walking I had done since I went blind 13 years earlier.[22] Let me tell you why, with the Orion, I could now do this.

---

[22] To watch a short video at this stage of me walking around my neighborhood, go to this link:

The thing about the Orion is that it gives the blind confidence to do things, to try things and to attempt new experiences. Confidence is the key here. Without confidence, you are not likely to try to do things. Indeed, you are nervous or maybe even outright scared. Before the Orion, I was too scared to walk around my neighborhood by myself, even with my cane. There were just too many things that were dangerous: obstacles in my way, inattentive car drivers, silent electric scooters speeding down the sidewalk, etc. The list is endless.[23]

Well, the Orion solves many of these problems simply because it gives the blind an added tool. More than that, it gives the blind confidence. Many speak of the importance of things like "independence" or "quality of life" that the blind lack, and which the Orion can increase. Yes, this is true. But, before all that, and more importantly, the Orion results in increased confidence. Confidence is the *sine qua non* to many, many things in life.

The Rehab Magnet Board, pictured at the beginning of this chapter, is a great training tool. It is about 20 inches wide by 17 inches high. One side is black, and the other side is white. To

---

https://www.dropbox.com/s/h0wlw69se35u1jg/WalkingWithOrion.mp4?raw=1

[23] I will not go into it here, but suffice it to say that it is amazing how unaware most people are of their surroundings. Even with cane in-hand and wearing my "blindman glasses," I have nearly been run-over by distracted car drivers, been shouted at by pedestrians for not moving out of *their* way while they walked down the sidewalk towards me and on and on and on.

maximize contrast, magnets of the opposite color (e.g., white magnets for the black side) can be placed onto it. These magnets come in all sorts of different shapes and sizes (e.g., squares, triangles, rectangles, strips, semicircles, etc.).

I spend about 15 minutes a day gazing at the rehab magnet board.[24] With my bionic eye, I look alternately at these various shapes. What I see as a particular shape is not what you see as that shape. For example, a triangle to me does not actually look at all how it looks to you. But, it does look triangle-like. The same goes for other shapes. They do not look to me how they look to you. However, the critical thing is that to me all of these shapes look different one from the other. I feel that somehow my brain will figure-out some way to recognize patterns.

A little further below, I tell the story of the radar scope operator in the Korean War. That story and the above expresses what is meant by learning to see with bionic vision. It is a process of learning to recognize things for what they really are based on how they appear to me, not how they appear to normally sighted people. This process is not easy or fast. It is, however, very challenging and exciting!

---

[24] Scientists who study the brain and the phenomena of neural plasticity say that about 15 minutes of brain-training is optimal. Doing more or less than that amount of training is not productive. To foster the re-wiring of the brain, about 15 minutes of training is best.

The Six-Month Evaluation

In December 2018, I had my six-month evaluation. It was now time to evaluate how things were going. The evaluation would consist of two different types of assessments. The first assessment would be a Functional Low-Vision Observer Rated Assessment (FLORA). The second assessment would be a battery of tests in the bionic lab.

Basically, the FLORA involves a trained, independent person coming to someone's home to observe how that person does things in their daily life with their very low vision. It assesses how the person adapts to using low vision aids to perform daily life tasks. FLORA is not specific to the Orion, but it turns-out to be an excellent way to objectively measure the effectiveness of the Orion in improving how its users adapt with it. After all, the Orion is a vision aid just like any other like reading glasses.

The FLORA specialists are not the same as the Second Sight rehab specialists mentioned in the previous chapter. Instead, FLORA specialists objectively *measure* how well the Orion user is adapting to the Orion. On the other hand, a Second Sight rehab specialist *trains* the Orion user in how best to use it. The point of a FLORA specialist is to determine the usefulness of the Orion to the user.

A lot of the time spent with the FLORA specialist is devoted to just talking about how I feel emotionally about the Orion. Besides all the quantitative measurements about the usefulness of the Orion, there is also an emotional impact that it has on the individual. A FLORA specialist makes an assessment of this too. You can surely imagine the devastating emotional impact on someone who loses their eyesight. What is less commonly known is that this happens in reverse too. That is, there is an emotional impact on individuals who regain eyesight.

I think it is fair to say that the impact of losing eyesight is nearly always negative, meaning it is depressing. That last statement makes you want to say "duh." You are not wrong. However, when someone *regains* eyesight it can go either way. That is, it can be a happy thing or a depressing thing. This needs a bit more explanation.

I am not going to go deeply into the emotional impact of regaining sight here. That is outside the scope of this book. A great deal has been written about this topic elsewhere.[25] Let me just say that I suppose that the main thing in determining whether happiness or depression results from regaining sight is what expectations the individual has about the nature of the "sight" they may regain. For example, in my situation I had a clear understanding about

---

[25] See, for example, the section about the psychology of vision restoration in the article "New Research Explained: Restoring Vision Following Long-Term Blindness: Prosthetic Vision and Considerations for Rehabilitation" at this link:
https://www.visionaware.org/blog/visionaware-blog/new-research-explained-restoring-vision-following-long-term-blindness-prosthetic-vision-and-considerations-for-rehabilitation/12

the Orion's rudimentary, synthetic vision. I had no expectation that I would have vision anything like what normally sighted people see. If I had, I would not be happy with its results. Simply put, my expectations were reasonable.

One last thing should be mentioned about the emotional impact on regaining sight. Surprisingly, there is an impact on those around the individual who regains some sight. And, there is an impact on personal relationships between, for example, a husband and wife or a boyfriend and girlfriend. Again, this impact can go either way. It can be either a positive or a negative thing. Some people may not like an increased level of independence that an individual who has regained some sight gets. They may then feel like they are less needed. On the other hand, some people may relish now being able to share visual things with the person who has regained some sight. Here, I will just say that everyone within the world of an individual who regains sight is impacted in one way or another. Countless things could be written on this topic alone.

So, for me, it is fair to say that at this early stage my FLORA results are wonderful! To me, my results are better than expected. I mean that both quantitively and emotionally. Of course, my assessment here is not scientifically or clinically measured. This is just how I feel about it. At the end of this chapter, I will explain why I feel this way and some of the astounding things I can already do.

Contrary to the FLORA assessment, the assessment in the bionic lab was a controlled, measured, scientific test of my vision. Essentially, it consisted of re-taking the baseline test described earlier in chapter 4 in the section about remarkable happenings in the bionic lab. Those three tests were the Square Localization, the Grading Visual Acuity and the Direction of Motion tests. For the assessment in the bionic lab, I took each of these three tests both *with* and *without* using the Orion. Then, those results were compared to when I first took these baseline tests before being implanted with the Orion.

When taking these baseline tests, how well you score on each is mathematically calculated in a very precise way. During this six-month evaluation, with the Orion I basically scored twice as good as I did when I first took the baseline test before being implanted. Not surprisingly, my score without using the Orion was essentially the same as it was before being implanted. This is an amazing thing. It is scientific evidence that, in fact, the Orion is working. And, for me it is working better than what might have been expected!

Over all, when thinking about this six-month evaluation and the Orion trial, I am frankly and happily a little surprised at the results. First of all, I am very glad simply to be alive and well - mentally and physically. Remembering just what this is - the first-ever human trial of a brain implant to create synthetic vision - anything could have happened. After all, at this stage, this whole thing is a test just to see if the thing is safe. That it is working as well as it is gratuitous.

One thing about the Orion is that different people will have varying results using it. At the six-month stage, Second Sight reported this variability. [26] Some users will do better than others. I am lucky in that, seemingly, my results are towards the high end of the scale. Although it is somewhat mysterious exactly what causes the variability in Orion results among its users, one thing for sure is that the person using it must be actively engaged in adapting to it.

Learning to see with the Orion does not come automatically. It is sort of like the difference between driving a high performance, stick-shift car like a Porsche versus hopping in the backseat of a self-driving car. The Porsche requires you to be very actively engaged to make it do its thing. You need to learn the fine points of operating a high-performance machine. On the other hand, for a self-driving car, you just jump-in and say "take me somewhere." If you merely turn-on the Orion and say "make me see" you may get a certain level of results. However, if you turn-on the Orion and vigorously train, adapt and exercise it your results will likely be better.

That the results with the Orion vary among its users is not surprising. It is, after all, a medical device. Everyone using any sort of a

---

[26] See Second Sight's press release dated January 7 2019 "Second Sight Reports Fourth Quarter 2018 Business Update" here: http://investors.secondsight.com/news-releases/news-release-details/second-sight-reports-fourth-quarter-2018-business-update

medical device will have varying results. For example, imagine you gave 100 of the exact same wheelchairs to 100 disabled people who all have the exact same sort of disability. Some of them would play basketball. Others would have difficulty just making it down the block. More than anything, I suspect that a person's degree of motivation and power of belief accounts for most of the variability.

Getting to Know My Bionic Vision

From the above discussion about the Rehab Magnet Board, let me explain some more about what my bionic, synthetic vision is like. Earlier, I explained that it is all in my mind's eye, and that it is a lot like a 1960s era, monochrome air traffic controller's radar scope. So, I must learn to *interpret* what I see. That is, I do not see images like how normally sighted people see them. Instead, I see an image that I learn to *recognize* as being something. This is best explained by a little story Mickey, a Second Sight rehab specialists, told me one day in the bionic lab about an Airforce radar operator during the Korean War in the mid-1950s.

During the Korean War, there were US Airforce bases located in Korea. Periodically, enemy warplanes would make attacks against these bases. One day at a particular base, the radar operator there sounded the alarm that there was an incoming attack by enemy warplanes. Because of this radar operator's early warning, many lives were saved. Soldiers had time to take cover. US warplanes had time to get protection.

For many years since then, and until the present day, as a training tool US military radar operators are shown the film of what was displayed on the radar scope during this incident. Everyone looks at the film and says that they do not see anything noteworthy, let alone something that might be an incoming attack by enemy warplanes. Only after they are pointed to a particular image appearing very faintly, and only in two-dimensional monochrome, do they then see that there is *something* there. In disbelief, everyone then proclaims that there is no way that this vague radar image could be identified as incoming enemy warplanes.

Afterwards, a film of an interview with the radar operator on duty this day during the Korean War is shown to the trainees. The radar operator is asked how he could have possibly not only seen something on his scope but known it to be an incoming attack by enemy warplanes. He answered very plainly, like it was a stupid question. He explained that he is highly trained, skilled and experienced at his job. He said that he has been watching radar scopes for so long that he can see *everything*. He said that he can tell an enemy plane from a friendly plane and that he can notice things appearing on the radar scope that others might not detect at all. Essentially, he has learned to interpret what he sees on his radar scope and, thus, can see what others might never see.

And so it is with my bionic, synthetic vision. I am like this radar operator from the Korean War. I do not see things the way *you* see things. Indeed, I see things very differently. But, I am learning to know instinctively what these images are that magically appear in my radar scope!

I am asked all the time by strangers, friends, family and scientists to describe what I see. This is a difficult thing to do. Only analogies can be used. Of course, having once had eyesight I can describe things in terms familiar to others. So, when I say that my bionic vision looks a lot like a monochrome radar scope - it really does. Sometimes, I wish you could see it for yourself. Oh well, I suppose you just have to trust me!

The Big Picture is the Little Things

I could rattle-off here a long list of things that I can already do because of the Orion, even at this early stage. However, the big picture is the little things. What I mean is that the fundamental thing, the big picture, is that there are things that I can do now that I could not do before the Orion. It is not so important precisely how well I see them. Most meaningful to me is how I *feel* about the things I can do. These are the little things. You can visit my webpage at richardbmcdonald.com where I blog about the evolution of my bionic vision. For now, the following tales about candles and the Super Blood Wolf moon expresses this somewhat.

One night in early December 2018, my wife Charina cooked-up some fish in the kitchen for dinner.[27] Naturally, cooking fish stinks-up the house a bit. So, as she usually does, Charina lit a scented candle in the kitchen. An hour or so later after finishing dinner I said to Charina, "Sweetheart, you better go blow-out the candle."

Charina declared to me, "**YOU** go blow-out the candle."

"Oh my God," I thought to myself! "Maybe, just maybe, I could." I was, after all, wearing the Orion device at that moment.

So, with some reservations about whether I would be able to do it, I walked into our kitchen. I knew the candle was there *somewhere*. I could smell it. To give me a better chance of seeing it, I turned-off the kitchen lights so as to improve the contrast the candle might make in the dark. Then, I began to scan around the kitchen with my bionic eye.

"Ping, ping, ping" went my bionic eye radar scope in a very particular area atop the kitchen stove. "Could it be the candle" I thought? Nothing else in the kitchen was triggering blips on my bionic eye's scope so much. I approached the source of the ping, leaned over a little, and nervously blew.

Do you know the smell a candle makes when it is first blown-out? Glorious! And, there was no more pinging in my bionic eye's radar scope in that particular area atop the kitchen stove. I did it! To see a candle and blow it out may seem a small thing to some people, but

---

[27] It tasted fantastic, Sweetheart!

many have said to me that it is stunning. I think so too. Ponder for yourself the following statement: a blind person was able to see and blow-out a candle. This might be called a miracle! If nothing else, the statement is an oxymoron.

Most meaningful, though, is what the little tale of the candle means for me. Guess what I get to do now? Blow-out my birthday cake candles! And, just like everyone else, I get to make a birthday wish! I have not been able to do this since I lost my eyesight 13 years ago. To be honest, I have always felt a little sad at birthday parties when the person blows-out their candles and makes a wish knowing that I cannot really do that. Now I can. See for yourself, as follows.

I wish you could have been with me one night in early 2019. It was my first birthday after getting bionic vision. My wife, Charina, and I went to a little Japanese restaurant for dinner to celebrate. After dinner, I was served a small cup of green tea ice-cream. It had one small birthday candle burning in it. I was wearing the device, the Orion. Several of the Japanese waitresses began to sing "Happy Birthday" to me. After everyone finished singing, it was time for me to blow-out my birthday candle and make a wish. The entire restaurant went silent. Everyone was holding their breath.

Using the device and scanning for the lit candle, I saw it. "Ping, ping, ping," went my bionic vision radar scope. I began to reach out with my finger towards the source of the pinging, asking in bewilderment if that was the candle? The Japanese waitresses cried -out in unison "No!" and grabbed my hand for I was moving my finger straight into the candle's flame.

So, with a big breath and an earnest wish, I blew at the flickering image caused by the Orion in my mind's eye. Suddenly, the flickering stopped. I did it! I then cried a little, for this was the first time I could do such a thing since I lost my eyesight 13 years ago. My wife cried A LOT, for this was the first time she had seen me do this for 13 years. All the waitresses cried out "HURRAY" in stunned amazement. Dozens of patrons dining at that moment who were aware of the unbelievable thing I was wearing - the Orion - witnessed the whole thing. All together, they shouted "Oh my God!" I want the world to know that a miracle happened this night inside a little Japanese restaurant in Los Angeles.

And now let me tell you that I, a blind man, saw the Super Blood Wolf moon.[28] On Sunday the 20th of January, 2019, there was a Super Blood Wolf moon in Los Angeles. I had

---

[28] It is a "super" moon because the moon is closer to the earth than usual, causing it to be noticeably bigger and brighter. A "blood" moon means a lunar eclipse that happens at nighttime, causing the moon to turn a blood-red color. This was also a full lunar eclipse. It is a "wolf" moon which means the first full moon in January. Hence, this was a Super Blood Wolf moon. See this link: https://www.space.com/43062-super-blood-moon-2019-last-until-2021.html

dinner at "Moonshadows" in Malibu that evening.[29]

At around 9:15 PM when the moon was at full eclipse, my wife Charina and I stepped out onto Moonshadows' deck. Gazing up into the night sky and scanning with the Orion, I could detect in a particular spot a VERY faint glint. It looked to me how a match might look to a normally sighted person at night from a city block away (~600 feet). Pointing to this particular spot in the sky, I asked my wife "Is that the Super Blood Wolf moon sweetheart?"

"Yes," Charina gasped!

I did it! I saw the Super Blood Wolf moon! Glorious! A Round of drinks on me was had by all that night on the deck at Moonshadows under the Super Blood Wolf moon.

No doubt, I am today full of pride, excitement and most importantly hope. I am proud to be in this clinical trial of the Orion, knowing that I am pioneering a wonderful thing for mankind. I am excited by the wonderous things that happen to me, like seeing candles and Super Blood Wolf moons. And, for sure, I dream about what I may see as the years roll-on.

---

[29] Moonshadows is, in my obviously biased opinion, the most wonderful restaurant in the whole wide world. From the age of about five continuing until the present day, I have had dinner there regularly. For the first approximately 35 of these years, I could see. And then, for about the next 12 years I could not. Now, with the Orion, I can. My wife, Charina, and I had our wedding reception there. If you are curious, see Moonshadows' website here: http://www.moonshadowsmalibu.com/

I often think about what those who come after me may see someday.

Yes, I am a little bit scared too. After all, nobody really knows yet just how far all this may go. And, things could go badly. But, so far so good! Most of all, though, no doubt I am a happier person today.

This Page Intentionally Left Blank

Chapter 7 - the Ethics of Bionics

Getting a brain implant for bionic vision immediately brings-up all the many issues regarding its ethics. It may come of a surprise but, to a lesser or greater degree, in fact bionics has been around for a long time. Really, it is nothing new. Of course, there are many ethical and societal considerations involved when thinking about merging humans with machines. However, upon reflection, it is a bit odd to realize that most of these ethical issues were settled some time ago.

From Captain Hook in <u>Peter Pan</u> (1904) to Tony Stark in <u>Iron man</u> (2008), bionics has come a long way. Of course, while Iron Man represents a bionic force for good, the dark side of bionics (at least initially) is represented by Arnold Schwarzenegger in <u>The Terminator</u> (1984). As usual, like nearly all technological advancements such as the Internet, there are both good and bad things that bionics bring with it.

It turns-out that the field of bionics is way further advanced than what is commonly known. I will talk a bit more about this in the final chapter of this book regarding the future of bionic vision. Suffice it to say for now that within 20 years from today, frequently meeting someone with bionic parts will not be an uncommon thing. Actually, it will become ordinary.

Whether or not any particular individual agrees with *how* these ethical issues have been settled is a different question altogether. Generally, bionics refers to the replacement of a body part with a mechanical substitution. Bionics are generally divided into two categories. The first category are bionics that simply restore a lost or broken body function. The second category are bionics that are meant to enhance a perfectly fine or otherwise unbroken body function.

Bionics are Already Here

Since ancient times, sundials had engraved on them various mottos. A very popular motto was "It's later than you think." This is very true when considering how far along bionics have come. It is a mistake to think that bionics are some distant thing that may or may not become a reality. They are already with us. It is later than you think.

Perhaps the most startling thing of all is just how fast bionics are coming into the ordinary world. For example, in chapter 4, I spoke about meeting Michelle Armenta Salas.[30] She is one of the Second Sight scientists working with me on the Orion. In that chapter, I talked about how shocked I was to learn that countless universities, like her *alma mater*, already offer Ph.D. programs in brain-machine interfacing (also called brain-computer interfacing or BCI).

---

[30] See also the Acknowledgements section for more about Michelle.

I did not know that bionics was so commonplace that Ph.D. programs are already offered at many universities around the world.

There is little disagreement about bionics that merely restore a lost or broken body function. However, sometimes the difference between restorative versus enhancement bionics is not so clear. Often, reasonable people will disagree about whether a particular bionic replacement is just meant to fix a broken function or instead intended to make-better an otherwise normal function. But, just where exactly is this line?

Usually, a bionic part is obviously meant just to fix a broken body part. Take for example the artificial heart. The first implantation of a modern artificial heart was performed in 1982 (the Jarvik artificial heart). Today, the technology and usefulness of artificial hearts is vastly better than it was in 1982. No doubt, an artificial, mechanical heart is a bionic restoration. Worldwide, there are thousands of people alive because of them. All reasonable people would say that this use of bionics is intended simply to fix a broken body part.

Bionics are a bit different from a simple prosthesis in that they match the original function more closely, or in some way improve on it. Obviously, crutches are not bionics. On the other hand, some modern examples of restorative bionics include Michael Chorost, who wrote a book about his personal experience with the cochlear implant (bionic ear) entitled <u>Rebuilt: How Becoming Part Computer Made Me More Human</u>. Does not that book title say it all? And then there is Jesse Sullivan, who got a robotic limb controlled by a nerve-muscle graph that allowed him a full range of motion far beyond a simple prosthetic. There are endless even more basic examples of what can be called bionic restorations, such as pacemakers.

Some might argue that for something to be "bionic" it must have some electronics in it. They might also argue that the bionic part must be implanted for it to be a real bionic part. I am not so sure this is true. To me, I think that these distinctions are not really all that important. The most important thing to me seems to be that the replacement or additional part mimics or improves on the original body function. That said, this is certainly a blurry line.

A good example of the blurry line that separates something that is not bionics from something that is certainly bionics involves the condition of sleep apnea.[31] This sleep breathing medical condition is most often treated with a continuous positive airway pressure (CPAP) machine.   A CPAP machine is not bionics. However, sleep apnea can now also be treated with an implantable device called Inspire.[32] The Inspire is an implantable device that delivers electrical impulses that cause the patient's airway to remain open while sleeping, allowing for normal breathing. It was approved by the

---

[31] See this Wikipedia article for more about sleep apnea: https://en.wikipedia.org/wiki/Sleep_apnea

[32] For the FDA's approval announcement about Inspire, see this link:
https://www.accessdata.fda.gov/scripts/cdrh/cfdocs/cfpma/pma.cfm?id=P130008

FDA in 2014. To me, the Inspire is an example of bionics. That said, it could be argued that it is not.

An interesting thing to notice about bionics is illustrated by this blurry line between a CPAP machine and the Inspire device. Notice that the former is an external device while the latter is implanted. That is, the Inspire cannot be removed or simply taken off its user. This is a hallmark of a bionic device. Although not a hard rule, generally speaking for something to be truly a bionic device it becomes an inseparable part of the body.

The preceding paragraph brings-up another curious aspect about bionics. Often, at first a device is something external to the body, then it becomes something worn by its user and finally something that is implanted into the body. In other words, it gets closer and closer to the body, ultimately becoming a part of it. For example, consider the iPhone. Presently, the vast majority of people just hold their phone external to their body. But now, you can wear an iWatch on your body. The next step is for cellular (i.e., "smart") technology to be implanted directly into the body. How long do you think it will be before that happens? In fact, it is already in the experimental phase.[33] Experts predict it will be a reality by 2023. Remember, it is later than you think!

---

[33] See this 2016 CNET article "The Mobile Phone of the Future will be Implanted in Your Head": https://www.cnet.com/news/the-mobile-phone-of-the-future-will-be-implanted-in-your-head/

One particularly quarrelsome area of bionics is the arena of sports. In 2016, the first Olympics involving people with clearly bionic body parts were held in Zurich, Switzerland. "Cybathlon 2016" (Cyborg Athlon) were the first Olympics for people with bionic body parts. Teams of people with various disabilities used bionics to turn themselves into athletes using things like powered prosthetic legs, robotic exoskeletons (like Iron Man) and motorized wheelchairs. The next Cybathlon is scheduled for 2020.[34] Although Cybathlon may not be so controversial because everyone competing has some bionics, what about the true and remarkable story about the "blade runner."

Oscar Pistorius was a 26-year-old South African athlete who competed in the 2012 London Summer Olympics.[35] He is often called the "blade runner." Oscar has artificial legs. At the age of one, both his legs were amputated below the knees. He became the first double amputee to compete at the Olympic Games. Oscar ran in the 100, 200 and 400 meter Sprints. To be clear, these events were in the *regular* Olympics, not the Paralympics.

Although sports competition officials at first objected to Oscar competing with "normal" athletes saying that his artificial legs gave him

---

[34] See the Wikipedia article about Cybathlon here: https://en.wikipedia.org/wiki/Cybathlon
[35] For purposes of the topic here, we will not get into Oscar's troubles later in his life. Suffice it to say only that several years after his Olympic competition Oscar was convicted in South Africa of murdering his girlfriend.

an unfair advantage, eventually they threw-in the towel. Maybe his legs are not true bionic legs, but they are certainly far more than simple prosthetics.[36] So, how far away or different is Oscar from an athlete competing in Cybathlon? Is it fair for humans without any bionics to compete in sports with those that have bionic parts? At what point does someone with bionics cross-over from being a human into being a cyborg? Will humans compete in sports against cyborgs? These ethical questions about sports and bionics are not settled.

Bionics are becoming Commonplace

Society's perspective on the ethics of bionics are changing rapidly. A fascinating example of this is how the different generations view bionics. In the next chapter, I discuss this a bit. While there is almost no ethical debate about bionics meant merely to restore a broken or lost body function, there is a lot of ethical disagreement concerning bionics meant to enhance or improve an otherwise normal function. That said, society's perspective about enhancing our bodies just because we want to for reasons of vanity or the desire to somehow be "better" than we were before is changing rapidly. It is fast becoming normal.

Consider as a simple example society's perspective on Plastic surgery. True, on the one

---

[36] To see a bit more about how Oscar's artificial legs work, see the Wikipedia article here: https://en.wikipedia.org/wiki/Mechanics_of_Oscar_Pistorius%27s_running_blades

hand, no doubt plastic surgery in the common sense is not really bionics. However, on the other hand, as a culture we decided long ago that there is nothing unacceptable about wanting to have plastic surgery to enhance ourselves in some way simply because we want to look better, to turn-back the effects of aging or to be seen as somehow "better" than others. There is every reason to believe that enhancing ourselves with bionics will be viewed culturally no differently than we view plastic surgery today.

Both men and women get all variety of plastic surgery for reasons of pure vanity. Men get hair transplants to turn-back the effects of aging on their loss of hair. Women get breast augmentation for reasons like wanting their clothing to look better on them. Hollywood is flooded with all sorts of plastic surgery. There is no negative cultural implication with any of this. Either men or women can, for example, get pectoral or breast implants simply because they desire the perceived enhancement to their appearance. They do this not for any medical reason due to a loss of body function caused by disease, injury or birth abnormality but, rather, just because they want to make themselves look better.

Even in what some may consider to be far out examples of plastic surgery, society has very little remaining negative bias. Actually, culturally this is most often envied and celebrated. Take as an example Kim Kardashian's rumored butt cheek implants. Since I have been blind for the past 13 years, really I do not know how her rear end looks.

However, I am told that it is a sight to behold! For the record, Kim denies getting butt implants. Others say she did. The point here is not the wonder and awe of Kim's butt but, instead, the majority belief of society today that it is perfectly fine if she did get butt implants.

Getting truly bionic implants is really only a very small step forward from plastic surgery. Undoubtedly, people will get bionic implants for purely enhancement reasons. That is, they will get them not to restore a broken or lost body function but, instead, simply because they believe the bionic implant will somehow make them better. As the availability and use of purely enhancing bionics becomes increasingly widespread, of course there will at first be some level of distaste. However, over time it will become acceptable, normal and eventually commonplace. This trend can already be seen.

Today, we can see the first hints at this societal trend with everyone desperately seeking the latest iPhone, the latest Tesla car and so on. It is not so hard to see a societal divergence between the "haves" and the "have nots." That is, those who have bionic enhancements are very likely to view those who do not have bionic enhancements as inferior to them. And why would they not? After all, those with bionic enhancements will actually really be faster, smarter, stronger or "better" in all sorts of ways. It is not likely that being "all natural" or "organic" will been seen as being better than being bionicly enhanced. Those with plastic surgery enhancements think of themselves as better looking than those without enhancements. Those with the latest iPhone look-down on those with an older iPhone model.

Going even further, there is the Transhumanist Movement.[37] They believe that bionic technologies should be vigorously exploited to improve humans. They support advancing all such technologies to address human conditions such as aging, disease and other human limitations. In fact, Transhumanists proclaim that bionics should be used to improve human speed, strength, endurance and intelligence. Those opposed to Transhumanists believe that their view leads to a society where purely human beings are considered to be somehow inferior to bionic beings. The opponents go on to say that Transhumanism leads to an endless pursuit of upgrades, updates and more and more bionic implantation.

The societal divergence between those with and those without bionic enhancements will be further accelerated by the unavoidable issue of having the money to pay for their bionic enhancements. Those with plenty of money, the wealthy, will get bionic enhancements whenever they want them. In the same way that the wealthy get plastic surgery, they will desire to upgrade themselves, prolong their lives or otherwise better themselves. Since money is not an issue for them, as a class of people the

---

[37] See this Wikipedia article for more about Transhumanism:
https://en.wikipedia.org/wiki/Transhumanism

wealthy will become further set apart by increasingly enhancing themselves with bionics.

For regular people with modest or even lesser financial means, bionics will not be readily available. As with all new medical advancements, initially medical insurance will not cover those costs. Generally, if ever, new medical advancements take years before they become approved by medical insurance. And, for many regular people, they do not even have medical insurance. What is worse for regular people is that even if medical insurance might cover a particular bionic part it would certainly only be in the case of a "medical necessity." That is, they would only get the bionic part if they somehow became injured (like a severely damaged leg) or lost some body function (like eyesight).

The wealthy do not have any of the limitations on getting bionics as do regular people. They can get them whenever they want. They can get them purely for enhancement reasons as opposed to the case of a medical necessity. Just like the wealthy might today get plastic surgery for no reason other than they want to make themselves somehow better, so will they seek bionic enhancements. Perhaps the greatest and unavoidable ethical issue regarding bionics is the societal divergence it will bring about between those with and those without bionics.

This Page Intentionally Left Blank

Chapter 8 - The Future of Bionic Vision

I am always fascinated by how the different generations think about bionic vision.[38] The way that the various generations think about this sort of technology says a lot about the future of it. Even more interesting is how the different generations view bionic technology socially. In the previous chapter, I spoke a bit about the ethics of bionics. There is a spectrum as you move from the older to the younger generations in their level of acceptance of bionics. The older generations think it all somewhat unnatural or even "unholy." The younger generations are perfectly comfortable with all of it. "No judgement," Generation Z would say.

Most curious is Generation Z (born after 2000). For Generation Z, these young people are not in the least surprised by bionic vision. To them, it all seems unremarkable and no big deal. Whenever I speak with Generation Z people about my bionic vision, they are a little bored with it. They appear to want to say, "Duh, hasn't this been around for a while already?" I suspect that the grandchildren of Gen Z'ers may see bionic vision become really good. For Generation Z, getting bionic vision will be rather

[38] The age ranges for the various generations differs a bit depending on who you ask. Here, I am rounding them based on how Wikipedia defines them. See the Wikipedia article here: https://en.wikipedia.org/wiki/Generation

routine. It will become about as significant as when nowadays people get plastic surgery. That is, it will be no big deal. I will talk a bit more about this later in this chapter.

The Millennials (born 1985 - 2000) think bionic vision is totally awesome! Sometimes, I am a little embarrassed when wearing the Orion in public because it looks a little freaky. This is not at all the case for the Millennials. They think it is really cool. I have a feeling that they *like* to be seen with me in public wearing the Orion. Maybe, for them, it is sort of like showing-off the newest iPhone.

However, the technology does not surprise the Millennials so much. For them, it is like bionic vision are to-be-expected. They think that bionic vision is about as innovative and extraordinary as the newest iPhone. For them, they seem to want to say, "OMG, like, what took them so long to make it?" One thing about the Millennials, more so than any other generation, is that they show great compassion and a real desire to become involved with bionic technology. Being as steeped in technology as they are, no doubt they are the future of bionic everything.

For my own generation, Generation X (born 1965 - 1985), we are amazed by the technology. As kids in the 1970s, we grew-up watching the TV show <u>The Six Million Dollar Man</u>. So, we all thought bionic vision was at least possible. The typical reaction from a Gen X'er is something like, "WOW, they did it!" We do not have much trouble believing that bionic vision is a reality today. Most, but not all, of the people in the present trial of the Orion (like me) are Gen X'ers. We are the pioneers.

And then there are the Baby Boomers (born 1945 - 1965). These are the people who conceived what bionic vision (and hearing, limbs, etc.) has become today. And yet, most of them seem not to believe that it really exists. Only when they see it with their own eyes do they believe it. Typically, their reaction to it is, "No way!" Unless the particular Baby Boomer happens to be some sort of a scientist or doctor, most often they have a difficult time believing that it is a reality. Usually, when I am wearing the Orion and speaking with a Baby Boomer they gaze at me in stunned amazement.

Finally, there are those from the Silent Generation (born 1925 - 1945). Now, these people *do not* believe it. Even when I am standing in front of them wearing the Orion trying to explain it, they just shake their heads and walk away in bewilderment. In fact, often they gasp somewhat in horror that it is unnatural, "unholy" or some kind of extra-terrestrial technology. Since they are mostly speechless about bionic vision, I cannot say what their typical reaction to it is other than, well, silence!

And so, from the perspective of my generation (Generation X), I can look back two generations to the Baby Boomers and the Silent Generation and forward two generations to the Millennials and Generation Z. There is a very apparent trend across the generations towards bionics becoming normal. This trend is not only towards the social acceptance of bionics but also

95

towards the reality of its technology. The technology has moved from the impossible stuff of dreams to the everyday occurrence. Of course, bionic technology did not magically appear today. Surprisingly, bionic vision technology goes back many decades.

The Origins of Bionic Vision

There are reports going all the way back to World War I (ending in 1918) of soldiers who had injuries to their head and were then stimulated with electricity. Those crude experiments, reportedly, did cause a simple visual response. However, the first modern, medical experiments began in the 1970s. A seminal article about early modern work on bionic vision was a 2002 Wired magazine article entitled "Vision Quest."[39]

In 1978, a patient was implanted with a stimulator on his brain. This was done just before the FDA outlawed human experiments on bionic vision in the United States. The patient, "Jerry," had dozens of wires coming out of the back of his head. Those wires were permanently imbedded through his skull into his brain. At a distance, it looked like he had a ponytail. He would be plugged into a computer seven feet tall, 10 feet wide and weighing two tons. The video stream from the camera (like a 1980s era VHS camcorder) would be processed through the computer, and then sent from the

---

[39] This article can be found online at this link: https://www.wired.com/2002/09/vision/

computer into Jerry's brain. The system was not portable nor wireless, to say the least. But, Jerry could detect light and other crude things.

Next came "Patient Alpha." He was implanted with a brain stimulator in 2001. Since the FDA still had its ban in place at that time, the surgery was done in Portugal. However, testing of the computer technology used with his implant was done within the United States. His system was, by the standards of the day, considered portable. Today, we would not think of Alpha's system as really being very portable. Basically, his system consisted of something like a gunslinger's pistol holster tied around his waist. One side held the battery pack, and the other side held the video processing unit. The camera was more like a helmet camera.

Alpha's system was not wireless, though. He still had wires coming out of the back of his head. But, unlike Jerry, these wires could at least be unplugged from tiny connections permanently imbedded into the back of his head. By this time, the technology had improved considerably as compared to Jerry's. Alpha could, for example, see a telephone across from him on a table.

A great leap came around 2013 with the Argus, discussed earlier in Chapter 2 where I describe the Orion. Although the Argus is the predecessor of the Orion, I think that the Argus can still be considered "early work." On the other hand, the Orion crosses-over into the present-day state of the art. There is one fundamental difference between the Argus and the Orion that causes this cross-over: the Argus is implanted into the eye and needs an otherwise functional eye and optic nerve, whereas the Orion is implanted into the brain not needing any function of the eye itself. This single difference between the two makes their potential use vastly different. Whereas the Argus is limited in its potential use, the use of the Orion is potentially unlimited.

There are other early-work systems than those discussed above. All of these systems are considered "early work" for a number of reasons. One main reason is their limited computer processing capabilities. Certainly, this applies to the devices up until the Argus and the Orion. And, even the Argus and the Orion in their present state want for increased computer processing capabilities. We will talk about this a bit more in the next section. So, although it is a somewhat blurry line, it seems that the Orion is the cross-over point into present-day bionic vision.

Present-day Bionic Vision

In late 2018, the editors of <u>Popular Science</u> magazine published a book called "Your New Brain, When Humans & Computers Merge." Notice that the question is no longer "if" but only "when," as stated in this book's title. With the Orion, this has in fact happened. You can see it for yourself in the picture on this book's cover. I have an implant in my brain. My brain has merged with computers to create synthetic, bionic vision. Julius Caesar would say, "We have crossed the Rubicon."[40]

So, with the Orion, a few fundamental things have developed. First, it is implanted directly into the brain making the underlying cause of blindness irrelevant. Next, it is portable. Critically, it is wireless. Lastly, the computer processing power had reached the point where it is adequate. These fundamental advancements with the Orion mark the cross-over point from early work into present-day technologies as they relate to bionic vision.

Notice that I say above that the computer processing power is "adequate." What I presently have I refer-to as "Orion 1.0." As described throughout this book, the real magic of the Orion happens in the Video Processing Unit (VPU). When talking about the VPU, specifically what is meant is the microprocessor and the software that it runs (today we call software an "app"). As advanced as Orion 1.0 is, it is only *just* adequate enough to handle the heavy computer processing power requirements needed to convert a video stream from the camera into electrical signals that the brain can interpret. Put another way, Orion 1.0 is somewhat limited by its computer processing power.

The camera I use with Orion 1.0 is not super fantastic either. It is an analog camera. The camera is a lot like an early 2000s era

---

[40] See this Wikipedia webpage for the gravity of what this phrase is meant to impart:
https://en.wikipedia.org/wiki/Crossing_the_Rubicon

webcam. Analog cameras are lousy in low-light or nighttime conditions. What is even more critical is that a tremendous amount of additional computer processing could be done if the video stream were digital versus analog. Of course, a digital video stream and all that additional processing would require even more computer processing power. The difference between what an analog versus a digital camera can do is like comparing a 1980s cell phone to an Apple iPhone X.

Over all, as far-out as Orion 1.0 computer and camera technology is, it is basically about 15 years old. That is, its technology is dated to around 2004. Now, it would be a mistake to think that this is some kind of a disappointment. It is not. For one thing, the central purpose of this clinical trial of Orion is to make sure that it is safe. Remember the Hippocratic Oath - first do no harm. One great thing too is that the brain implant does not need to be "upgraded." As the external hardware of the Orion (i.e., the VPU and the camera) advances, it is designed to be compatible with the existing implant. Fantastic advances will come to the Orion as new external hardware is developed.[41]

---

[41] Of course, eventually the technologies related to the brain implant will advance. That will mean that at some point in the future people will get a better implant. And, some day the technologies related to the external hardware (the VPU and the video camera) will advance to a point where it is not compatible with my implant. However, this is not the case for Orion 2.0, and I suspect Orion 3.0 (discussed later) will very likely also be compatible with my implant.

Orion 2.0 is thought to become available sometime in 2020. Among other advancements, it will have a much more powerful VPU (microprocessor). It will also have a digital video camera. Naturally, as it is with all advancements in technology, it will be smaller and lighter. And, Orion 2.0 might even be a bit more stylish! As it is now, my Orion 1.0 is not gorgeous looking.

I have spent some time discussing above the external hardware (the VPU and the video camera) and the brain implant of the Orion. However, perhaps more important than that is the Orion's software, or the app. The app runs on the VPU translating the video stream from the camera into electrical signals that are sent to the brain implant. Those signals are then interpreted by the brain as synthetic, bionic vision. As such, the most important thing in the Orion is the app. That is where the real magic happens. So, really what the app does is to convert the video stream into a language that the brain understands.

Writing the computer code of the app is an enormous project. Essentially, it requires a deep understanding of the language of the brain. To put it into relative perspective, and this is only my personal wild guess, I suspect that in my lifetime the quality of the app in terms of the synthetic vision it can produce may progress a bit past the stage of DOS (1980s era PC software). The Millennials may see the app's technology reach the stage of Microsoft Windows 95. As for Generation Z, well, by the end of their lifetimes I suspect that they may have an app whose relative quality is beyond today's Windows 10. Their technology will employ AI and VR (both discussed below). Of course, predicting things like this are very difficult. On the one hand, it has taken decades to reach the point where we are today. On the other hand, the advancements are happening at an ever-increasing pace.

One thing is for sure - these advancements in the technology of the app will require ever-increasing computer processing power. For example, you could not run Windows 10 without great trouble on a typical PC built before around 2008. They simply would not have the processing power. The great news is that this required computer processing power does, and will, exist. And, the video camera technology does, and will, exist. The greater the computer processing power is, the more that can be done by the app. Plus, the better and "cleaner" the video stream is, the more that the app can do with it to create synthetic, bionic vision.[42]

---

[42] It is a bit technical and perhaps beyond the scope of this book, but a word about computer processing power and video should be mentioned. Doing simple computer tasks like working on a spreadsheet, writing a document or making a Facebook post requires only a small amount of power. On the other hand, processing video requires an enormous amount of power. Furthermore, the Orion is processing video 100% of the time. In comparison, for example, when someone takes a picture or a video clip with their smart phone its microprocessor is working only for a brief moment. Even more, the Orion is not just simply processing the video like how a smart phone does. It is additionally running all the algorithms to

I can make a few educated guesses today about what Orion 3.0 may look like. Beyond that, it falls into the next section about the future of bionic vision. Orion 3.0 may, at a guess, become available around 2023. Its external hardware will, at a guess, be twice as powerful as it will be in Orion 2.0. The state of the app by then will no doubt be advanced from where it is today, but how far it may be advanced is unknown. Also increasingly involved at this stage will be the as-of-now unknown mysteries of the brain itself and how it takes to all of this. Earlier in this book, I described the factors that determine the quality of what is seen. These will all be in-play with Orion 3.0.

Second Sight has mentioned additional technologies it is presently working on. Among those technologies are eye-tracking and object recognition capabilities. Eye-tracking would allow someone with the Orion to see something on their periphery by turning their eyes towards it without moving their head. This is how normally sighted people look at things. Object recognition capabilities would use technologies like facial recognition algorithms to synthetically enhance raw images as they stream through the Orion into the user's vision. Other things like books, phones, utensils, fire extinguishers and an endless list of other objects may be recognized too.

In addition to the above-mentioned technologies that may be incorporated into

---

convert that video into the language of the brain and transmit it wirelessly to the brain.

Orion 3.0, there may also be things like thermal imaging. Second Sight is presently working on this and the above-mentioned technologies.[43] Remarkably, once a good link between the Orion's camera and brain implant is established, a whole host of currently off-the-shelf technologies can be relatively easily plugged-in. Besides thermal imaging, night vision, zoom, ultraviolet and many other modes could be made available. It is not hard to see a day where, for example, an Orion user is walking around at night and switches to night vision to see better - and maybe even better than those without the Orion! None of this is beyond imagination today.

What the Future of Bionic Vision Holds

In the near-term future of bionic vision, say out until 2025, there are advancements that can definitely be seen coming soon. In the preceding section, I have described the advancements in terms of Orion 1.0 (what I have now), Orion 2.0 (perhaps in 2020) and Orion 3.0 (my guess is 2023). So, for discussion purposes, we can say that Orion 4.0 may come out in 2025. That is where the near-term future begins.

---

[43] See Second Sight's press release dated March 13, 2019, "Second Sight Reports Fourth Quarter and Full Year 2018 Financial Results" at this link:
https://www.businesswire.com/news/home/201903130 05801/en/Sight-Reports-Fourth-Quarter-Full-Year-2018

I should also say here that as I use the terms Orion 4.0, 5.0 and so on I do not necessarily mean the actual Orion device. As described in the following paragraphs, there is work being done by dozens of institutions all around the world on bionic vision. So, what I really mean is Orion-like devices.

Naturally, as anyone tries to predict technological advancements, such predictions rapidly become increasingly inaccurate. The good thing is that the advancements tend to come faster, but often in ways that were not predicted. For example, Thomas Watson (the chairman of IBM) said in 1943, "I think there is a world market for maybe five computers." Not counting mainframe computers and only counting smart phones and PCs, today there are billions of computers in the world. "We will never make a 32-bit [Windows] operating system," Bill Gates (the chairman of Microsoft) said at the launch of MSX in 1983. Windows 1.0 would not be released for another two years in 1985. It was essentially a front-end to DOS which was an 8-bit operating system. The laptop on which I am writing this book runs the 64-bit version of Windows 7. So, no doubt whatever happens in the future with bionic vision it is likely to happen faster and in ways that cannot be foreseen today. Nonetheless, some near-term, broad certainties can be foreseen.

It is not too hard to imagine the vast amount of technologies used by self-driving cars being incorporated into the Orion. For sure, there are two specific technologies that will have a massive near-term impact on bionic vision: artificial intelligence (AI) and virtual reality (VR). Like everything else, undoubtedly bionic vision will be connected to the Internet. And, the medical, surgical and materials sciences advancements will make present-day methods seem barbaric.

AI is likely to have the soonest impact. Some beginnings of it may come into Orion 4.0. For example, Soroush Niketeghad has written, "A visual prosthetic BCI [brain-computer interface]in its simplest form maps the light intensities in the visual field [from the camera] to [stimulate] the [brain]. Incorporation of [AI] into the BCI could potentially improve the device performance in different ways. [One] approach being developed is using [AI] for image processing to produce visual perception optimized for the specific task in hand such as navigation or face detection."[44] In other words, AI can be incorporated into the app (discussed in the preceding section) to greatly improve the translation of what is viewed by the camera and then transmitted to the brain. Basically, AI can intuitively "know" what is being viewed by the Orion's camera. Then, it can employ the best techniques to translate that image into brain stimulation that causes the best image in the mind's eye of the Orion's user.

---

[44] You can read his entire paper "Brain Machine Interfaces For Vision Restoration: The Current State of Cortical Visual Prosthetics" at this link: https://www.dropbox.com/s/vjpprbi0igrtn7e/BrainMac hineInterfacesForVisionRestorationTheCurrentStateOfC orticalVisualProsthetics%20%20.pdf?dl=1

VR will likely come into the Orion in the near future, perhaps around Orion 4.0. That technology could do some stunning things. For example, it is not too difficult to imagine VR enhancing the incoming video stream so that it appears better to the Orion user. Remembering that what is seen with the Orion is like a mono chrome radar scope, now think of a black-and-white movie (B&W). VR could take an incoming video stream, make it B&W, then make the darker things darker and the lighter things lighter and finally outline everything in very bright lines. This would improve everything's contrast and definition, thereby making the Orion user's vision much more useful. The possibilities with VR technology are endless.

Of course, like everything else, one day soon the Orion will be wirelessly connected to the Internet. With that, the possibilities are boundless. For example, it could use facial recognition technology and cross-reference that with your Facebook page and alert the Orion's user to the presence of one of your "friends." That same technology could likewise identify, as a small example, a photograph, an image on a screen or the physical presence of every popular individual (living or not) - celebrities, historical figures, politicians, uniformed policemen and firemen and so on. The Orion user could have an account "in the cloud" where they upload pictures of all their co-workers, their pets or anything else. Ultimately, perhaps in Orion 5.0, I do not see any reason why everything on the Internet could not be streamed directly into the Orion user's mind's eye. Imagine your smart phone's screen right in your mind's eye. Why not?

The medical, surgical and materials sciences involved with the Orion will continue to advance in fantastic ways. As an example, in 1960 the first heart bypass surgery was performed. However, since 2001 the number of these types of surgeries has declined by more than 50%. This is because of the advances in medical and surgical methods used to treat heart conditions today (e.g., pharmaceuticals, stents, etc.).[45] The biocompatible materials and fabrication methods (let alone the computer technology) used to make my Orion brain implant did not exist 20 years ago. No doubt, 20 years from now (2039), the medical, surgical and materials sciences then will make today's sciences seem like the work of witchdoctors.

Naturally, all of these foregoing near-term technologies will be integrated and synergetic. There will be vast advancements in these technologies that will make the Orion into something hard to imagine today. And, there will be new technologies developed used by the Orion that do not exist today and that cannot even be imagined. It is just like what is said in the introduction to the 1970s TV show <u>The Six Million Dollar Man</u>, "We have the technology. ... Better, faster, stronger."[46]

---

45 See this Wikipedia article:
https://en.wikipedia.org/wiki/Coronary_artery_bypass_surgery
46 See this YouTube link for this introduction clip:
https://www.youtube.com/watch?v=HoLsoV8T5AA

Work is presently being done that will revolutionize bionic vision in the long-term future (say, beyond 2030). It is likely that high-resolution bionic vision may be realized. In 2017, the Defense Advanced Research Projects Agency (DARPA) funded several institutions to make this happen. DARPA calls this project the Neural Engineering System Design (NESD). On DARPA's website, you can read their post entitled "Towards a High-Resolution, Implantable Neural Interface."[47] DARPA says there that they have specifically designed this project to make its discoveries commercially available. Seemingly, this work would result in very high-quality bionic vision.

In addition to the above NESD project, DARPA is also funding a futuristic project at Columbia University in New York. In 2017, DARPA made a $16 million grant to Ken Shepard to fund his work at Columbia. Ken is an electrical engineering Professor. He previously worked for IBM designing microchips. Professor Shepard's work intends to create a brain implant similar to the Orion, but with orders of magnitude higher resolution. Professor Shepard said, "What we're trying to do is extraordinarily ambitious, but I really think we can build this. It doesn't violate any laws of physics. This is absolutely doable from where we are now."[48]

---

[47] See DARPA's website post here:
https://www.darpa.mil/news-events/2017-07-10
[48] See the article "Brain Implants May Be the Answer to Restoring Sight" on Columbia's website at:

DARPA and its collaborators are far from the only ones working on the long-term future of bionic vision. In Europe, there is the Cortical Visual Neuroprosthesis for the Blind project; which aims to demonstrate the feasibility of a cortical neuroprosthesis interfaced with the visual cortex. Back in the US, there is the Utah Electrode Array project; which is beginning to test the "Moran/Cortivis Visual Prosthesis." Down under in Australia, there is the Monash Vision Group. Their work may result in a brain implant with resolution many times higher than what is available presently. This is only a small listing of the work being done worldwide with the goal of creating high resolution bionic vision. If we could know today what the long-term future of bionic vision will be, we would think it is magic.

Way out in the long-term future is the concept of tapping into the brain's ability to generate "sight" when dreaming. Think for a moment about what you see when you dream. What you "see" is entirely created with your mind. It is in color and has depth and resolution far greater than the best 4K Ultra HDTVs today. So, the brain has the ability to generate "vision" all by itself without any signals from the eyes whatsoever. Therefore, if science can crack the code about just how to translate a video stream and then transmit that to the brain, vision as good as what normally sighted people see can be synthesized. Does that seem crazy? Well,

---

https://news.columbia.edu/content/Brain-Implants-May-Be-the-Answer-to-Restoring-Sight

ponder the work being done right now described in the preceding few paragraphs. Now, ask yourself what the next level after that will be.

My Bionic Vision Future

For me personally, I suspect I may get to use technologies through Orion 3.0 or maybe 4.0 (as described in the preceding section). By then, the technologies will probably move beyond what my brain implant can handle. Put another way, at some point my brain implant will not be backwards compatible. Earlier in this book, I talked about why I did it; that is, why I decided to participate in this first-ever human clinical trial of a brain implant for bionic vision. One of those reasons was that, in balancing my age, health and other factors, out to around Orion 3.0 is about as far as I thought I could go.

But then again, in reality nobody knows just how far even my technology will go. There are factors at play here that are not well-understood today. The power of the brain and neural plasticity are great unknowns. And, the future technologies alone will do things that cannot be imagined today.

You can take this journey together with me. I have a blog at richardbmcdonald.com. There, I will post all about how this all goes. Whatever happens, it is going to be absolutely wild, fantastic and stunning! Ozzy Osborne said it best in his song *I don't know* "Nobody ever told me, I found out for myself. You've gotta believe in foolish miracles."

Acknowledgments

Second Sight Medical Products, Inc.: Second Sight was born out of the Alfred E. Mann Foundation (AMF). AMF is based on the belief that, although fantastic research is done in universities, hardly ever does it make its way into things that help the public. Its mission statement is, "To develop and commercialize innovative solutions for significantly unmet or poorly met medical conditions." Essentially, the AMF brings together the smartest people on the planet and grants them whatever resources are needed to solve medical conditions that the rest of humanity thinks are unsolvable or that are not commercially viable. You may have heard of an earlier AMF creation: the cochlear implant (made by AMF's spin-out company, Advanced Bionics) which allows the deaf to hear. To all the brilliant people at Second Sight I express my warmest appreciation. You did it!

Nader Pouratian, M.D., Ph.D.; Associate Professor, UCLA Neurosurgery: Dr. Pouratian's primary neurosurgical interest is in surgeries that preserve and restore function to patients. He is particularly interested in studying brain mapping signals to develop brain-computer interfaces to help patients with severe disabilities. Dr. Pouratian is the Principal Investigator at the UCLA Neurosurgical Brain Mapping and Restoration Lab. Dr. Pouratian heads-up the Orion clinical trial at UCLA for bionic vision. He performed the brain implant on me. Because of his great skill and good hands, getting a brain implant was easy. Thank you, Doctor!

Uday Patel, Ph.D.; Senior Research Scientist, Second Sight Medical Products, Inc.: Uday received his Ph.D. in 2007 from the UCLA Neuro Sciences Inter Department Program. He has been with Second Sight for more than 10 years. Uday has devoted his entire career to bringing sight to the blind with bionic vision. He is among the deepest thinking persons I have ever met. Besides all this, Uday is a scholar and a gentleman. Uday's belief in and perseverance with these technologies as well as his personal sacrifices made along the way to further these technologies are to be commended.

Vara Wuyyuru; Senior Clinical Research Scientist, Second Sight Medical Products, Inc.: Vara received a Master's Degree in Biomedical Engineering from Louisiana Tech University. She did her undergraduate work at Osmania University, India; whose motto is (perhaps not so coincidently) "Lead us from Darkness to Light." Vara has authored numerous academic and scientific papers about artificial vision. I think that Second Sight has selected the brightest people from countries around the world to solve blindness. Vara is India's gift to humanity's quest for that cure. She has helped me tremendously to learn to see with the Orion.

Michelle Armenta Salas, Ph.D.; Research Scientist, Second Sight Medical

Products, Inc.: Michelle earned her Ph.D. from Arizona State University in Brain-Machine Interfacing (also called brain-computer interfacing). Prior to joining Second Sight, she was a postdoctoral scholar at California Institute of Technology (Cal Tech). At Cal Tech, her main area of work focused on, among other things, developing brain implants for paraplegic patients to control a robotic hand. Despite these astounding accomplishments, Michelle is young. She devotes many long hours, not to mention her astounding brain power, working to make bionic vision a reality. I believe that Michelle will solve many baffling mysteries about how vision and the brain works.

This Page Intentionally Left Blank

Appendix A - Questions I Had Before Deciding

Making a decision to volunteer into any clinical trial is a scary thing. When the trial is for a drug, it is one thing. However, when the trial is for the first-ever *brain implant* into humans for bionic vision, the fear-factor rises to a whole new level. So, I had many questions before making my decision. Those questions are below. Obviously, they were answered to my satisfaction since I did it. You can visit my website at richardbmcdonald.com where I blog about some of the issues raised by these questions. I also post there more generally about the evolution of my bionic vision.

1. What are the short- or near-term risks associated with the implant surgery, in general? For example, what risks are there for infection, discomfort or pain, headaches and so on?
2. Can I roll around in bed when sleeping following the surgery? That is, would the implant in my head cause any problems with how I sleep as regards the position of my head?
3. What are the long-term risks associated with the implant surgery, in general? For example, is there any potential for (or information regarding) physical changes that might be caused to the brain (e.g., memory, other senses like

hearing, etc.) or personality changes (e.g., one's sense of humor, one's taste in music, etc.) that can happen?

4. How big, and exactly where, is the hole that is drilled into my skull for the implant?

5. How long will my skull take to heal?

6. After healing and my skin and hair re-grows, will I still have some sort of a scar, hole or divot in my skull? Does the drilled-away bone re-grow, or is some sort of hard, artificial material placed there for protection? Put another way, after healing could I feel the implant itself under my skin?

7. Am I able to swim, bathe, shower and so on with the implant?

8. With the implant and after healing, am I able to participate in moderate exercise and sports activities like aerobics, Yoga, running, jumping, body-surfing and so on?

9. What is the useful life of the implant? Some implants do not always have a "lifetime" useful life (e.g., a dental crown, a hip replacement {at least the older ones}, etc.) and must, at some point, be replaced or removed.

10. After the five-year clinical trial, if I wanted to, could I have the implant removed solely at my discretion and for whatever reason? And, would this removal be fully paid-for by the trial?

11. At any point during the clinical trial, if I wanted to, could I have the implant

removed solely at my discretion and for whatever reason? And, would this removal be fully paid-for by the trial?

12. Suppose some medical issues arise that are associated with the implant or use of the device, will the clinical trial pay for any necessary medical care that I might need? How is this handled both a) during the trial and b) after the trial? As regards after the trial, for how long would I be covered?

13. At some point in the future, were an upgrade to the implant desirable could it be replaced and so upgraded? For example, suppose that a new, wholly different methodology is developed, would having this implant prevent me from getting any such new method?

14. What is the purpose of the "headband" component of the device? I understand the purpose of the device's other two components (i.e., the glasses and the video processing unit), but the purpose of the headband is a little unclear to me.

15. What is the transmission range of the device's processing unit to the implant? For example, instead of wearing the video processing unit under my shoulder, suppose I had it on a table ~10' away from me, am I still in-range?

16. As the technology relative to the device itself (i.e., the camera, the video processing unit, etc.; not the brain Implant) progresses, would I get such upgrades?

17. Could I leave the implant intact but not ever use the device after the study for the rest of my life and just not use it?
18. What are the risks (both with and without wearing the device) relative to the implant from, for example, operating my ham (a.k.a., amateur) radio including my hand-held radio, going through a metal detector like at the airport TSA screening, having a dental x-ray, getting an MRI or CAT Scan, standing near a microwave oven and similar electromagnetic interference? If such electromagnetic interference happens, would it cause me to see images or hallucinations?
19. What is Second Sight's level of commitment and expectations as regards continued development and investment in Orion?
20. Throughout the trial, what level and sort of support will I receive, and from whom? For example, would I take user support questions to UCLA or Second Sight? What about any technical or medical issues I may encounter with respect to my participation in the trial? To whom would I take any such issues?
21. After the conclusion of the trial, suppose I kept the implant. Can I keep the device? Would I receive ongoing support, and from whom and for what?
22. What happens should I keep the implant and the device after the trial ends, and at some time thereafter Second Sight is no

longer around? Who, then, would I turn
to for ongoing support and should any
technical or medical issues arise?

23. The first time someone turns on the
device, what's it like for them? This isn't
a technical question about what they
may (or may not) see, but more about
the emotional reaction they have. For
example, do they faint, get dizzy or get
nauseous?